MEDICAL SCIENCE AND MEDICAL INDUSTRY

MEDICAL SCIENCE AND MEDICAL INDUSTRY

The Formation of the American Pharmaceutical Industry

Jonathan Liebenau

The Johns Hopkins University Press
Baltimore

First published in 1987 by
The Johns Hopkins University Press,
701 West 40th Street, Baltimore, Maryland 21211

Consulting Editor in the History of Medicine: Caroline Hannaway

Library of Congress Cataloging-in-Publication Data

Liebenau, Jonathan.
Medical science and medical industry.

Bibliography: p.
1. Drug trade—United States—History. 2. Pharmaceutical policy—United
States—History. 3. Medical innovations—United States—History. I. Title.
II. Series. [DNLM: 1. Drug Industry—history—United States. 2. Technology,
Pharmaceutical—history—United States. QV 711 AA1 L7m]
HD9666.5.L54   1987   338.4'76151'0973   86-27346
ISBN 0-8018-3356-6

Contents

Preface

Since the late nineteenth century the pharmaceutical industry has been the most profitable major manufacturing sector. Drug companies have also been among the leaders in capitalisation, product innovation, research sponsorship, multinationalisation, export earnings, and numerous other areas. The industry has also had to withstand repeated attacks from critics within and outside the medical world.

The form the industry is in today was not fixed, as most people currently in business believe, just before the beginning of their working lives, but rather at the time when the relationships between product development and marketing were stabilised, between company size and organisation institutionalised potential for flexibility, and between therapeutic products and medical practice became accepted by medical practitioners. These relationships changed significantly after the Second World War, but the foundation on which they were built was, by that time, large enough and strong enough to accommodate the major transformations engendered by the introduction of new classes of drugs, a new scale of regulation, and a rapid acceleration in the pace of business internationally.

This industry has been much written about by economists, business studies experts and even political scientists. It has been under almost relentless attack since the late 1950s for a variety of sins, including market manipulation, price fixing, dumping and all manner of unethical medical and business practices. Some of these are evident even in the early history of the industry, but that is not the purpose of studying the development of pharmaceutical manufacturing. It seems more important to be able to show what the characteristics of the industry are, and therefore why certain behaviours might be expected. In general, the pharmaceutical industry has not acted differently from other industries operating in similar markets. I am not particularly interested in whether the industry behaves 'ethically' or 'morally'. I am not looking for cases which show how the industry withholds necessary products from key markets, or dumps substandard drugs on less wary customers, or cynically manipulates the prices of products which are relied upon for health or nutrition. This is the sort of behaviour of large and powerful industries, especially those which operate internationally and wield professional, economic and political power. We should not be shocked by this, or be so naive as to believe that it differs in kind from other industries. The significant difference, however, is that this industry associates itself with the high standards of the healing arts. It was industry image-makers who chose, long ago, to let people think it was especially ethical. They claimed to have standards and a moralistic stance higher than other industries. Similarly, they chose to market their products as part of the pure calling of high science. This they did partly because their competitors did, partly because they came to believe their own rhetoric, and partly because they found that it works well in advertising.

This book grew out of a longstanding interest in the character of science, technology and medicine in commerce. Focusing on the pharmaceutical industry proved the best way to combine these interests and brought me in touch with a large variety of other themes relating to the character of technical change, the growth of big business, and the relationship between therapeutic products and medical practice. With such a diversity of topics the importance of centring this study on the industry became vital for the sake of maintaining continuity and order. Besides, the industry is of great importance in its own right and has been used as an exemplar of many things in the business world.

Readers of this book will bring to it their own prejudices. Whatever their premise, however, I believe that a detailed history of a variety of aspects of the industry will do something to add to the understanding of an industry which enters the lives of most of us in a uniquely powerful way.

Acknowledgements

No history of an industry can be written without depending on the sources held in company archives. I am indebted to the many people who made it possible for me to work in private collections. These and other archives are listed at the end of this book, and each entry implies further debts to archivists, company historians, public relations officers, support staff and people who helped me to arrange research visits.

Libraries and librarians on both sides of the Atlantic were also necessary for this work. The initial research was done at the Library of the College of Physicians of Philadelphia and the National Library of Medicine, but other special collections, including the Wellcome Institute for the History of Medicine and the Royal College of Surgeons were important to me, as well as general libraries, especially the Library of Congress and the British Library.

This book began as a doctoral dissertation at the University of Pennsylvania and I acknowledge the valuable help of many teachers as well as fellow students. Charles E. Rosenberg, Rosemary Stevens, Thomas P. Hughes and Russell C. Maulitz especially deserve my sincere gratitude. Financial aid came in part from the Smithsonian Institution, where I was twice a fellow, and from the Pharmaceutical Manufacturers' Association, whose grant was generously given with no strings attached. Further support came from the Leverhulme Trust through the Business History Unit of London University. My former colleagues at the London School of Economics gave me tremendous encouragement and guidance.

JONATHAN LIEBENAU

1 Introduction: Medicine and Technology

The pharmaceutical industry has produced the majority of new medicines, as well as imaginative science and considerable profits since the nineteenth century.[1] Its close relationship with the medical community, which in the United States developed during the Progressive Era, was instrumental to this success, and changed the character of medical practice as much as it did the industry itself.[2] Despite the importance of the pharmaceutical manufacturers in the development of modern medicine, however, they have almost been ignored in standard medical history accounts.[3] When the commercial significance of medicine has been examined, it has usually been from the point of view of the economics of private practice, insurance and hospitals; not the companies.[4]

This book sets out, therefore, to examine the evolution of the pharmaceutical industry itself. Since the adoption of scientific techniques, or at least of a scientific veneer, seems to have been crucial to success among the drug companies, the relationship between science and the industry will form a central focus here. I shall analyse why firms embarked on 'research' in its broadest sense, as well as considering on a larger scale the forces influencing drug companies to innovate. General business forms were changing rapidly during the Progressive Era, with important implications for pharmaceutical companies.[5] But the drug industry changed far more radically as a result of alterations in the scientific and technical resources available to them.[6] Most importantly, these included such personnel as medical men, pharmacists, other scientific staff, as well as labourers who were amenable to the kind of exact, repetitive and standardised tasks which characterised drug production by the First World War.[7]

The years 1890–1930 are the focus here because it was during this period that medical manufacturing assumed its modern form. However, where previously studied, the history of pharmaceutical

1

manufacturing has been characterised as if the antibiotics and the psychoactive drugs introduced after the Second World War made the industry.[8] While the production of these drugs has promoted remarkable growth since the 1950s, the earlier history of the industry shows that the companies had already developed the structure upon which this later growth could be based. Moreover the industry had established a secure place within the medical community by the Second World War, a development which ensured a continuing – and profitable – partnership between producers and consumers.[9]

Though this book covers the industry nationally, there are certain local characteristics which have influenced the study. While New York city served as the centre of a large part of the wholesale trade, and midwestern firms such as Parke Davis in Detroit, Eli Lilly in Indianapolis, and Upjohn in Kalamazoo, were important, Philadelphia stands out especially. Leaders in all sectors of the industry were either based in the city, moved there during this period, or established facilities in the region for aspects of their business.[10] Individually, companies elsewhere were significant, but none formed part of a medical community in the way that the Philadelphia manufacturers did.[11] The pharmaceutical industry in Philadelphia serves two important historical functions that make it particularly worthy of study: it was a leading community in its own right, with considerable national influence, and it represented a pattern of development to be found elsewhere.[12] Moreover, Philadelphia provides a coherent geographic focus with a well-knit medical community. The city's physicians formed a nationally important medical group and their schools and associations were widely influential throughout the United States.[13] Philadelphia's medical industry, though large and diversified, was nevertheless an integral part of that community.

SCOPE

The organisation of this book emphasises the development of individual companies within an industrial and medical community.[14] It stresses how companies used scientific innovations and staff, and how they changed from nineteenth-century drug compounders into the large-scale producers and powerful institutions of the mid-twentieth century. In Chapter 2, there is an overview of the industry in the nineteenth century. Chapter 3 moves to a detailed study of companies and the medical community in the early 1890s. American practitioners were beginning to adopt medical science, at least in the leading urban academic institutions; a change which had profound implications for the pharmaceutical industry. Meanwhile, businesses were shifting towards a departmentalised management structure which was to favour the inclusion of the newly popular scientific work.

Focusing on the production and use of diphtheria antitoxin, Chapter 4 discusses the particular significance of antitoxins in bringing public health and hygiene movements into the sphere of scientific medicine, and from there to pharmaceutical manufacturing itself.[15] Although city and state public health departments were the first to undertake the production of diphtheria antitoxin, the drug companies soon responded to the challenge, seeking to eclipse government ventures. The antitoxins and related biologically produced medicines (in contrast to extracted or compounded drugs) forced the transformation of the medical industry. Commercial production of these drugs brought the H. K. Mulford Company into prominence, as described in Chapter 5. The style set by Mulford and its main competitor, Parke Davis and Company, became a major factor in changing the marketing of drugs into a battle for scientific credibility. In the following chapter, the impact of the introduction of science on the whole of the medical industry is examined in an overview of pharmaceutical production up to the First World War. Laboratories were used in a variety of ways as scientists searched for appropriate roles and companies applied them to a range of business problems.[16] Some trained pharmacologists and physicians were used, for example, almost exclusively to defend companies when medical expertise seemed a useful legal tool; others were employed in a perhaps more predictable way, to expand product lines by developing new drugs or by copying from competitors. Chapter 7 analyses the effects of government intervention on the industry after Congress enacted regulations in 1902 requiring licences for the producers of biologicals. This law, and the more famous 1906 Food and Drugs Act, were in part responses to such leaders of the industry as Mulford and Smith Kline for more stringent technical standards which gave them clear advantages over competitors with poorer laboratories.

During the First World War, the army bought large quantities of medicines, bringing further prosperity to companies which had already achieved considerable success through selling vaccines to municipal public health departments. The war was also a watershed of a different kind. Since the 1890s, German chemical companies had been applying a concerted strategy to control their American markets by holding United

States patents. During the hostilities these monopolies were broken. Chapter 8 discusses the case of the antisyphilitic, Salvarsan '606', with respect to the efforts of the Dermatological Research Laboratories to produce the drug in the United States after 1916, thereby violating German-held patents. The problems they encountered were typical of such patent evasion. The first difficulty was in reproducing the drug – no mean feat when the inventor, Paul Ehrlich who worked in cooperation with the Hoechst company in Frankfurt, was the only consistently successful producer. They then had to surmount the legal barriers of the Hoechst patent and an exclusive licensing agreement with the influential New York chemical importer, Herman A. Metz. Finally, the Dermatological Research Laboratories had to prove its own reputation in order to sell its product. The concluding chapter brings earlier themes together in an analysis of the American pharmaceutical industry up to the Great Depression. During this post-war period, scientific research became institutionalised throughout the industry; it had become a necessity if a firm were to maintain a scientific image and remain competitive in the market for sophisticated products. Control of product quality and the satisfaction of standards set both by the government and the medical community also became increasingly important.

TRENDS

As pharmaceutical firms grew from apothecary shops to family companies and then to large corporations, their relationship with the medical community also changed. Pharmacists held a tenuous place in the medical world of nineteenth-century America, although they provided important services to those members of the public who did not use physicians, and supplied those who did with medicines.[17] Towards the end of the century drug makers distanced themselves from pharmacists and their informal practice of medicine. As the distinction between reputable manufacturers who sought the professional market – 'ethical' pharmaceutical producers – and the popular 'patent medicine' makers grew,[18] the large companies looked for a compromise between the two areas. They hoped to establish reputations for quality but also to reap the profits from patent or proprietary medicines. Adapting to developments in scientific medicine, by the 1890s many of the leading companies were projecting a new and avowedly scientific image: they began to employ medical men and maintain laboratories for quality control, standardisation and, in some cases, product development.[19] These small laboratories gradually evolved into significant research and development facilities which by the First World War were supplying new products to a medical world newly insistent on novel scientific therapies.[20]

The pharmaceutical industry changed both quantitatively and qualitatively between 1890 and 1930.[21] Its growth remains a central question for historical explanation. Since few have sought to elucidate the industry as a whole, this question has barely been addressed. An exception is William Becker who, in a 1969 study of hardware and drug wholesaling during the second half of the nineteenth century, gives four reasons for the growth of large-scale manufacturing of pharmaceuticals. Innovations in methods of drug preparation allowed factories to use machinery, and the growth in popularity of standardised preparations permitted new economies of scale. Becker further cites changes in therapy and the influence of research conducted in the companies as other causes of the industry's expansion.[22]

Becker's analysis stresses characteristics of the drug industry which address issues of particular concern to economic historians.[23] Though incomplete, it is a starting point for further discussion. The use of machinery, for example, enabled E. R. Squibb and Eli Lilly to secure large government contracts for basic drugs such as opium, quinine and ergot during the Civil War.[24] Fast-operating tableting machines, like the ones patented in 1890 by Oberlin Smith and Abraham Morris and assigned to H. K. Mulford, were examples of one aspect of large-scale production.[25] Innovations of this type were certainly advantageous for those few manufacturers who, like Squibb, could afford to invest in a large production plant and who felt that their market was sufficiently stable for them to predict consumption patterns.[26] Collaboration with manufacturing chemists was also important in leading to the use of machinery, particularly in Philadelphia where such prominent chemical companies as Rosengarten and Sons provided local models of large-scale production and technical expertise.[27]

However, small-scale producers were by no means defeated after Reconstruction by their lack of mass-production capabilities. As late as 1890, a number of pharmacists were still increasing their production in order to enter the wholesale market. As long as they held at least one assured market they were able to survive competition from large manufacturers.[28] Moreover, early efforts to develop new drugs and production processes even in the larger companies were not 'research', but rather the routine recombination of accepted remedies into new products.[29] Investment in research or large-scale manufacturing did not become a competitive advantage for most firms until well after the passage of the Pure Food and Drugs Act of 1906.[30]

Physicians increasingly relied on pharmacopoeiae, a trend that encouraged the growth of a market for standard preparations and, conversely, a smaller one for apothecary-compounded drugs.[31] Apothecary practice also changed because visiting salesman began to deliver orders frequently and this, together with increasingly reliable transport, meant that pharmacies began to stock smaller quantities of drugs.[32] Changes in therapy towards more specific drugs with measured doses also encouraged the introduction of the standard preparations produced by companies.[33]

These shifts in the industry, however, do not adequately explain its expansion around the turn of the century. A limited conception of research in the companies is particularly misleading, especially if it leads to the assumption that there was a constant level of reasonably sophisticated analysis and invention throughout the late nineteenth century.[34] Science played another and far more important role: with its ability to alter a firm's image, it became a major tool for expansion, permitting companies to grow in parallel to their counterparts in other industries.[35]

The term 'science' was used by the companies in an all-embracing manner. We can break it down and speak of the two most important aspects for them. The first was the form of science, both in conceptual content and in laboratory procedure.[36] Scientific activity became experimental on a large scale at the end of the nineteenth century, moving from its seventeenth-century image as an empirical, rational body of knowledge. The experimental science of the nineteenth century required laboratories with specific hardware and a staff organised around particular projects.[37] When this form of scientific activity was first adopted by drug companies it was quickly taken beyond an earlier natural philosophy approach of collecting new herbs and classifying them according to therapeutic effect.[38] The new 'science' was progressivist and explanatory in its claims.[39] Furthermore, it promised to control nature by curing disease, even to the extent of ending epidemics.[40] However, early work in the new industrial laboratories established procedures for testing, measuring, standardising, analysing and synthesising; original research followed later only in a few companies. Such research was less important – despite the impression often given by the companies and later historians – than the more routine applications of scientific technique.[41]

The second important aspect of 'science' at this time was its image. Companies deliberately exploited their association with science, with all that it promised in the public mind. Scientific medicine seemed to hold new power from the end of the nineteenth century: bodily functions suddenly appeared explicable and diseases curable, according to the novel formulations of such disciplines as physiology, immunology or bacteriology.[42] Firms also addressed their scientific rhetoric to the medical community, which was itself increasingly using scientific language.[43] Neither of these uses of a scientific veneer had any necessary effect upon drug production; rather they served to associate companies with an image of advance, both in medical and lay eyes.

Drug companies began scientific research, therefore, for a variety of reasons. Some proprietors appear to have been interested in providing the public with new cures. Although this was probably not a major incentive for any company, it seems to have been a sincere concern for some employees.[44] Many companies saw a need for standardisation, or were forced to standardise by government regulation, and therefore employed a scientific and medical staff for the purpose.[45] Many were primarily concerned with the side-effects of having technically trained personnel and sought the advertising advantages that the association with a scientific image provided. In other cases, the need for liaison with the medical and academic communities was particularly important, especially for those companies at the forefront of development and marketing.[46]

The set of new approaches, techniques, teachings and interpretations of scientific medicine promised to transform not only the pharmaceutical industry but also medical practice. That promise manifested itself in revised prescribing patterns. Since drugs provided the most effective means for physicians to exercise their new therapeutic function as scientifically advanced practitioners, the pharmaceutical companies became increasingly central to the medical community.

The unique character of the 'prescription' drug market, in which patients had limited control over what they paid for and physicians carried a restricted responsibility for their medicines, encouraged the industry to concentrate on addressing the medical men. Although prescriptions were not required for patients to obtain most drugs during the period, manufacturers could choose to advertise certain products only to physicians. By controlling the information available to their customers, company scientists found themselves able strategically to use the image of science to promote their medicines. The image which the prescription drug manufacturers cultivated was that of a high-technology industry,[47] and was an image forcefully contrasted with that associated with the crude production methods of patent medicine makers.[48]

Patent remedies, usually used without a physician's guidance, had long been controversial. The work of scientists and technicians in the pharmaceutical industry forged a new link between organised research and the competitive marketplace. The techniques of vaccine and serum production were aggressively applied to a range of products after the stunning success of diphtheria antitoxin in the 1890s. Though many of these, such as a widely marketed antimeningitis serum, failed to work, their sophisticated means of production and the seeming elegance of the underlying theories swayed physicians.[49]

Companies also wished to distinguish their products from 'patent medicines', and found secrecy more effective than patents.[50] Moreover, American firms did not conceive of using patents in the strategic, all-embracing way in which the German chemical companies did.[51] The drug industry began to innovate significantly just before the war as new techniques bore fruit. Its research style, however, was unlike other industries. In contrast to the emergence of electrical manufacturers, for example, patents were little used by most American pharmaceutical firms until the mid-1920s.[52] Patenting was not an effective way to secure a monopoly, particularly as it was very difficult to show that a patent was unique and defensible, or to prove infringement. Hoechst routinely patented the chemical products of their scientists in the United States,[53] but when their employee, Emil Behring applied for a patent on diphtheria antitoxin his request was repeatedly denied by the American patent examiner on the grounds that it was not an original invention. Immune reactions had been noted before, the official argued.[54] Although in this case Behring was eventually successful, his experience shows the difficulties of acquiring patents for medicines under the operation of such criteria.

The industrial development of new science-based products created an impetus for institutionalising research. And this in turn helped to tie companies into the medical community more tightly than ever before. Institutional forms of research varied widely between firms. Some enterprises such as Parke Davis and Company and the H. K. Mulford Company built large research establishments by drawing from the medical community. Most hired a few medical scientists to provide them with the capabilities for standardising and testing, quality control and process adjustment.[55] Collaboration also varied widely. Some companies established formal associations with local universities or colleges of pharmacy. Parke Davis had early links with the University of Michigan, recruiting both students and faculty as well as funding studies.[56] Mulford maintained close ties with the Philadelphia College of Pharmacy, offering prizes to top students and providing facilities at the company for botanical and pharmacological research.[57] Herman Metz took advantage of a tenuous connection with Columbia University, while the scientists at the Dermatological Research Laboratories were all faculty members at the University of Pennsylvania.[58]

Associations with hospitals were less formal but at least as important.[59] Because most physicians worked at the company part-time they were usually involved in a variety of other professional jobs. Some taught at medical schools or worked in public health, most had some form of private practice, and many had hospital appointments. For them especially, hospitals provided the opportunity to use new remedies. This form of testing was informal and unchecked. But a successful trial at a major hospital would often be used in advertising a new remedy.[60]

Job mobility was high among the staff of drug firms throughout the period. Strategic moves boosted the careers of key people, especially technical personnel, for whom the currency of their trade was the novelty of their ideas and techniques.[61] This mobility served as an important means for transferring production techniques. Competitors often initiated new production lines after hiring knowledgeable people away from well-established firms. This form of transfer was in practice far more important for development than the literature readily available on particular medicines and their methods of production.[62]

A new relationship with employees of the federal government developed with the growth of drug regulation. Like other regulatory agencies, those responsible for the drug industry worked in close collaboration with the leading producers. The mobility of personnel among the companies, universities and regulators was representative of the 'revolving door' which has been a feature of government–industry relations since the Progressive Era.

What brought medical men to the companies when they usually had other career options? The companies paid well for their expertise.[63] They also provided equipment and support staff unavailable elsewhere. At a time when research facilities were not normally provided by universities, even in medical schools, the opportunity to work in a well-financed, modern laboratory was a major inducement for some. Firms presented an image which was strikingly employed by Sinclair

Lewis in his novel, *Martin Arrowsmith*: The Hunziker Company was an old and ethical house which:

> dealt only with reputable doctors – or practically only with reputable doctors. It furnished excellent antitoxins for diphtheria and tetanus, as well as the purest of official-looking labels on the swaggeringly modest brown bottles.[64]

Despite the scorn of his friends and colleagues, Arrowsmith's teacher, Max Gottlieb, was attracted to the excellent facilities, steady work and high pay offered by commercial laboratories:

> Gottlieb found such laboratories as he had never planned, and instead of student assistants he had an expert who himself had taught bacteriology, as well as three swift technicians, one of them German-trained . . . If they talked too much of money – of how their salaries would be increased – yet they were free of the careful pomposities of college instructors.[65]

To his fellow immunologists, Max had 'gone over to that damned pill-pedlar', and Martin shuddered to see the man he most respected 'falling for those crooks'.[66] But the temptations were great, and even Arrowsmith later found himself succumbing to the lures of a commercial laboratory.[67]

The study of the pharmaceutical industry can be placed into three distinct contexts. In relation to the history of medicine, it provides a perspective on the producers and manipulators of therapeutics. The medical industry also employed many physicians and medical scientists, whose influence on the companies themselves was as significant as the impact of the industry on medical practice. Second, the study sheds light on medicine as technique and technology.[68] The medical industry must be viewed, together with the hospital, as a major source of medical technology; it was also the originator of technique, in that it provided new therapies and devised methods by which to use them. Third, this work relates to literature in the history of technology and business on the development of new industrial sectors, of science-based industry, and the particular problems of marketing esoteric products to consumers who were ill-informed about the forefront of development.

2 The Development of the Pharmaceutical Industry, 1818–90

PHILADELPHIA DRUG MAKERS, 1818–40

The foundation for the pharmaceutical industry in the United States was laid in Philadelphia between 1818 and 1822 with the establishment of half a dozen enduring fine chemical manufacturers.[1] America had formerly been dependent on Britain for most of its medicines, as for other manufactured products. With the economic disorder created by the war of 1812 and its aftermath, this pattern of dependence was broken. Since importation was disrupted and high tariffs were levied on those goods which did get through, it became easier and more profitable to manufacture many products than to ship them from England.[2]

The production of most common medicines was within the reach of many apothecaries. There was little need for high capital investment, and only a general knowledge of pharmacy practice was necessary for them to produce such basic remedies as quinine sulphate, opium powders, or calomel.[3] Demand was constant and universal, and profits were temptingly high.[4] Americans were enthusiastic takers of remedies, as was noted by one foreign observer:

> The amount of medicine prescribed in a large city is prodigious, the estimate being that in New York alone at least a million and a half prescriptions are compounded annually. . . . How much of this is wasted on imaginary ills no statistics will ever inform us.[5]

The laboratories of many pharmacies could be turned into manufacturing plants. When Charles Ellis and Isaac P. Morris bought the Marshall Drug Store in Philadelphia in 1818, for example, they

11

expanded the laboratory to begin large-scale production. To do so they installed a boiler in the cellar, created a drying room for plants and marked out a storage area. They equipped themselves with a jacketed copper pan, a filter press and open furnaces.[6] With little more investment they were able to compete on the local wholesale market with major manufacturers and importers, making a full range of opiate preparations, herbals and materia medica. Such was their success that by 1850 they had accumulated sufficient capital to move into a factory building and abandon the retail business. Their move gave them the opportunity to introduce steam-driven stirring and grinding apparatus, further increasing their capacity.[7]

An operation on the limited scale of the Marshall drugstore could manufacture a wide variety of products, since the mechanical and chemical processes were basically similar for most preparations. The production of medicines lay midway between the manufacture of chemicals and the practice of pharmacy. Most drugs at the time were made by such basic processes as crushing, drying, extraction and distillation. For example, cloves were dried, crushed and powdered to produce a popular anaesthetic; and juice from belladonna plants was extracted and then distilled to concentrate it so that it could be used as a heart stimulant.[8] Analogous procedures were followed by chemical manufacturers to produce pigments, acids, sodas and other commonly-used substances. Pharmacists not only borrowed from the chemists in their procedures, they also overlapped in their products. The firm of John Shinn, Jr, for instance, manufactured calomel, vermillion, red precipitate, corrosive sublimate, cinnabar and some mercury preparations, as well as crystallised soda, aqua fortis, hydrochloric acid and other chemicals, thus supplying both industrial and medical needs.[9] The simplicity of procedures allowed considerable diversification, which in turn permitted the development of wide markets or the strategic use of particular product lines according to demand.

Foreign-trained pharmacists founded many of the new companies established in the second decade of the nineteenth century, and these firms came to dominate the American chemical and pharmaceutical industry into the twentieth century. One Englishman, John Farr, teamed up in 1818 with a Swiss pharmacist, Abraham Kunzi, to manufacture medicinal chemicals in Philadelphia.[10] Their success was assured when they introduced to the United States the profitable Seidlitz powders, a digestive medicine already popular throughout Europe.[11] They later became part of the firm of Rosengarten and Sons, which had developed into one of the world's largest chemical manufacturers by the end of the century. Its origin was the partnership of Seitler and Zeitler, two other immigrant pharmacists who set up shop in 1822.[12] They originally manufactured such basic medicinals as quinine sulphate, sulphuric ether and ammonia water, and by the 1830s offered a variety of preparations of morphine salts, mercurial drugs and strychnine.[13]

Drug use has always been associated to some extent with therapeutic theory, although less than is often thought.[14] In the early nineteenth century medicines were compounded and administered both by doctors and by pharmacists. Both patients and medical men identified the immediate and dramatic reactions caused by most drugs as part of the cure.[15] Competing in a crowded marketplace for patients,[16] as part of the cure doctors needed to demonstrate the efficacy of their treatments, and the remedies they prescribed were designed to cause easily perceptible changes in the physical state of the patient. Coupled with the mutual faith which physicians and patients had in these treatments, drastic remedies served to satisfy the demands of patients for effective cures.[17]

The basis of this faith was a coherent system of therapeutic theory. Charles Rosenberg has done much to delineate this system and to describe its function as an acceptable framework of explanation. He has suggested that beneath it lay the notion that the body was in a constant dynamic relationship with its environment. Equilibrium was associated with health, imbalance with disease, and the purpose of therapeutics was to restore order. Humoral theory and localistic models of disease were reconciled by the principle that every part of the body was related inextricably to every other. Rosenberg identifies the early nineteenth-century conception of the body as a system of intake and outgo.[18] Physicians and patients could see and judge excretions or appetite; they therefore seemed an obvious monitor of health. Therapy, as a result, concentrated on diet and excretion, perspiration and ventilation as the aspects which could be controlled to produce a stable system.[19]

If a person had a wound, for example, he or she might be treated with a salve locally, but the holistic implications for the body might well necessitate the administration of a stimulant in addition. Enormous quantities of medicines were consumed in order to maintain or re-establish health.[20] Special medicines were also administered in life crises, or at changes of season, when a patient's body was more liable to lose its healthy equilibrium. Cathartics, for example, were given in the spring and autumn to help the body adjust to these cyclical changes. Mercury treatments and bleeding were the most common severe therapies, both producing dramatic effects.[21]

This therapeutic framework was not necessarily interpreted by a physician: in the first half of the nineteenth century many Americans avoided doctors altogether and consulted pharmacists. Preference for self-dosing and the lesser expense of druggists stimulated trade in patent medicines.[22] These remedies, often standard preparations of common drugs sold by brand name or unusual concoctions of stimulants, alcohol and flavouring, sold exceedingly well. Most of the drug companies which originated in pharmacies or from wholesalers depended upon patent preparations for the bulk of their profits.[23]

The stocks of drugstores contained large selections of raw chemicals, herbal remedies, special preparations and proprietary medicines. The nature of the stock can be seen from an examination of the staples regularly carried by Philadelphia drugstores according to a mid-century assessment:

Drug staples[24]

arnica flowers
balsam peru
balsam tolu
bicarbonate of soda
blue vitriol
borax
canary seeds
cantharides (Russian and
   Chinese)
carbonate of ammonia
cardamon seeds
cassica
castor oil
chamomile flowers
cinchonidia sulphate
citric acid
cloves
cream of tartar crystals
ergot
essential oils
exalic acid

gum camphor
gum shellec
hemp seed
insect powder
iodine chlorate
ipecac root
jalop root
mercury
morphia
morphine
opium
potash: bichromate, bromide
prusiate
quinine
soap
squill
sugar of lead, white
tartaric acid
tonca beans
vanilla beans

Although this list lacks a number of standard preparations such as belladonna and well-known, if little used, herbs such as sarsaparilla and mandrake, it indicates the range and type of medicines employed before South American and African explorations yielded large numbers of tropical herbs.

Pharmacy as a retail business expanded rapidly in Philadelphia during the first half of the century often as a sideline to medical practice for physicians. One commentator complained that:

> Fifty-seven of the drugstores in Philadelphia were kept by physicians, who left them in the hands of medical apprentices or hired assistants. The competition among pharmacists in Philadelphia is so excessive as to be a chief obstacle to the attainment of a higher standard of knowledge and skill among them. There are retail stores in which the whole year's sales do not reach $1000, – and in most of them the annual receipts range from $1,500 to $2,000.[25]

Despite this involvement of physicians in the sale of drugs, medicine makers had a long tradition of strained ties with mainstream practitioners.[26] The United States differed, of course, from Great Britain where apothecaries had early formed a guild and had been in direct, open competition with doctors.[27] But even though the rift was never so wide or formalised in America, there was suspicion among some physicians about the extent to which pharmacists were actually diagnosing and prescribing.

There is much evidence to suggest that their suspicions were well-founded. Periodically the conflict would be raised in the medical literature or in state governments. In a comment about the shortcomings of a proposed law in the later nineteenth century, the *Medical Times and Gazette* made it clear that pharmacists had long encroached on regular physicians' preserves.[28] The journal noted that the new legislation still would not:

> prevent an apothecary from compounding and selling a remedy, or himself prescribing and making up his own prescriptions. . . .[29]

The nostrum makers who really tested the patience of physicians were those who used false medical credentials to promote their products. Dr Robertson's pills, for example, were the invention of so-called 'Dr' Thomas W. Dyott, a prosperous druggist who regularly misused such credentials. He had emigrated from England in 1806 and immediately set up a patent medicine business.[30] In 1810 he attached 'MD' to his name and within a few years had secured a large market producing 'Robertson's Infallible Worm Destroying Lozenges' and other proprietary medicines for sale all over the east coast.[31]

When it came to promoting drugs, patent medicine makers outstripped either pharmacists or 'ethical' pharmaceutical firms. They were masters of innovative and persuasive advertising, famous for elaborate graphics. In the Philadelphia area they could be seen flaunting their products from:

the walls of our inns – the corners of our streets, and our pumps thereof – the wrecks of burnt, dilapidated buildings, with their standing abutments – the fences enclosing vacant lots . . . and the decks and cabins of our steamboats.[32]

However much they may have been disparaged by regular medical practitioners and pharmaceutical firms, the latter were soon forced to follow their lead in advertising. Thomas Dyott's use of newspapers and regional agencies became a model for a number of other such manufacturers, and slowly spread throughout the industry generally.[33] By the 1830s his advertisements were to be found in local newspapers throughout the country and he had marketing agents in New York, Cincinnati, New Orleans and elsewhere.[34]

The period 1818–40 saw the establishment and steady growth of a number of small pharmaceutical firms in Philadelphia. Robert Shoemaker became perhaps the first large-scale manufacturer in the city in mid-century; his success was built on the production of glycerin. Shoemaker started his career with a retail pharmacy in 1836 but took every opportunity to mechanise. 'Rub! Rub! Rub! day after day, and yet the labor continued. Thankful may the modern apprentice be that this work is now [c.1880] done by machinery.'[35] His expansion in the 1850s into drug milling and wholesaling assured his financial success.[36]

Another company whose origins and operations were typical of this time was that of Smith, Kline and French. John K. Smith had come from Montgomery County, Pennsylvania, and acquired his licence as an apothecary in 1829.[37] In 1830 he set up business in the city with his brother-in-law, John Gilbert, establishing their shop at 296 North Second Street, in the middle of Philadelphia's most densely populated section. Smith and Gilbert divided the business in 1837 and Gilbert moved two blocks away to compete with his former partner.[38] The financial panic of 1837 seems to have added to Smith's good fortunes, drug-making being one of those businesses often able to withstand financial adversity.[39] The 1841 Philadelphia City Directory listed the business as that of John K. Smith and Company.[40] 'And Company' referred to a new partnership with his brother, George K., who took over the shop three years later when John died. John's widow and his brother became executors of his estate, for which they had to post a bond of $50 000, which gives an indication of his wealth.[41] By mid-century, as earlier suggested, a few firms were becoming particularly well-established.

EXPANSION AND THE CIVIL WAR YEARS, 1840–70

Philadelphia and New York were by this stage the main suppliers of drugs. They still concentrated on purchasing from London, while the London import–export merchants assembled chemicals, materia medica and medical equipment from all over the world.[42] Drugs were distributed in the United States through a marketing network which extended to all the rural general stores and physicians as well as the city pharmacies. Most medicines were sold by grocers or doctors, who stocked the drugs they were most likely to use.[43]

The activities of Troth and Company illustrate a typical operation before the Civil War.[44] Strong marketing techniques were needed to place firms in the forefront of competition, and Troth concentrated in particular on these. The firm provided a number of services to physicians in addition to stocking a full range of pharmacy products, mostly from foreign sources.[45] It drew upon the wide variety of retailers in Philadelphia who dealt with medical products, including publishers, to arrange for the purchase of books, prosthetics and teaching aids. It then supplied these as a special service to its favoured market, small merchants and established physicians in the west and south. Troth's customers included residents of central and western Pennsylvania, western Virginia, Tennessee, western Maryland, Ohio, Missouri, the Carolinas, Alabama, Mississippi, Georgia and Louisiana.[46]

To provide complete marketing services, the company arranged with forwarding and commission agents in Pittsburgh, Cincinnati and other western cities to transport their goods. To compete with other wholesalers the firm often paid freight rates to those cities. For sales where they were in direct competition with New York and Baltimore merchants, they discounted the differences in transport costs. Thus in 1843 when selling to Pritchard and Son in upstate New York, the firm paid 'all expenses on such of our goods as you may order, to New York [City], so as to place us on the same footing with you as the New York druggists';[47] and to a Maryland customer Samuel Troth explained: 'To compete with the Baltimore Druggists I have paid the freight on thy goods to that place.'[48]

Troth's method of competing through discounts was not the only means adopted by firms in their attempts to capture distant markets. At Smith Kline and Company, George K. Smith began to prepare precisely measured drugs for physicians, rather than the less accurate quantities mostly used by pharmacists. This practice helped to establish his reputation as a major supplier for physicians, and by the mid-1840s he was producing more drugs than he could sell in his immediate area. He sought to supply physicians at a more distant remove and soon received proof of his status when, during the war with Mexico (1846–48), he secured contracts with General Winfield Scott's troops for quinine, one of his major products.[49]

However, Smith lost his army contracts on the outbreak of the Civil War, as well as the trade that he had built up with southern and western customers.[50] His consequent business failure stands in contrast to the huge success other drug sellers found in the Civil War. E. R. Squibb for example secured his first massive sales during this time, building a reputation for being able to supply the forces in the first years of the war with high quality goods relatively promptly.[51] The Army Medical Department purchased large quantities of drugs as a response to fears of price fluctuations and lapses in supplies of imported drugs. The Philadelphia firm Wyeth and Brothers benefited particularly from the department's orders, selling $657 122.17-worth of chemicals, drugs and medical supplies.[52] Wyeth in turn purchased from other Philadelphia firms, including Henry Bower, and Powers and Weightman, to fill the army's orders.[53] Powers and Weightman was known for the quality of its ether, after a committee of the Boston Society for Medical Improvement found it superior to Squibb's renowned preparation, and anaesthetics were, of course, much needed during the war.[54] Powers and Weightman and their local competitor Rosengarten and Son were also the only firms who produced quinine in quantity before the war and, since imported drug prices reflected financial speculation during the hostilities, these Philadelphia companies became important sources of supply for the army.[55]

The unrestricted boom did not persist throughout the war. In 1863 Surgeon General William Alexander Hammond sent Assistant Surgeon Joseph H. Bill to assess Squibb's laboratory. Hammond wanted the army to manufacture its own medicines and hoped to learn from Squibb how best to do this. Squibb persuasively argued that his operation alone was capable of meeting most of the government's needs and that, in any case, the investment necessary for large-scale production was too large for the army to undertake on short notice.[56] Despite Bill's acceptance of this argument, Hammond pursued his scheme. Bill had learned sufficient from Squibb's laboratory for him to be able to direct one of two army chemical manufacturing laboratories established in 1864, virtually in competition with commercial manufacturers.[57] The two laboratories, one in Long Island and the other in a building in Philadelphia formerly owned by Powers and Weightman, produced a large proportion of the medical supplies which in the first half of the war had been bought on the open market.[58]

In balance the army laboratories did not greatly harm the private sector, since government production was offset by the increased demand for both patent and traditional medicines created by the war. Many firms, such as Rosengarten and Weightman,[59] prospered, although others, such as Smith Kline and Company, lost ground. But even the latter did not suffer long. George K. Smith was forced in 1863 to sell a large interest in his firm to George Y. Shoemaker, upon which the company was renamed Smith and Shoemaker. After the war the company was able to build anew with Shoemaker's investment. In 1868 it passed the $100 000 milestone in annual sales. Smith died that year and his nephew, Mahlon K. Smith, became general manager, ousted Shoemaker, and changed the firm's name to Mahlon K. Smith and Company.[60]

War conditions and good prices encouraged pharmacists to produce on a larger scale. Many over-extended themselves and the decline in the market after 1867 left those producers and wholesalers over-capitalised. As they unloaded their stocks, prices fell even further, marking the beginning of a decline in the wholesale drug price index which lasted almost to the end of the century.[61] Pharmacists reacted to the reduction in profits from their drug business by stocking a wider variety of prepared medicines and branching out to carry such 'fancy goods' as brushes and mirrors, candy and cleaning items.[62]

A comparison of the 1860 and 1870 censuses of manufacturers in Philadelphia shows the over-all growth of the pharmaceutical industry over the decade. The number of establishments manufacturing medicines, extracts and drugs rose from 173 to 292 and the number employed in them more than quadrupled, from 1059 to 4729, while capital investment grew even more, from $1 977 385 to $12 750 809.[63] Since pharmaceutical manufacturers used wholesalers to distribute their drugs, the wholesale price index allows us to assess the over-all fortunes of the drug trade in relation to the economy as a whole, as measured by the index for all commodities.[64] Although drugs were aggregated with chemical products in the statistics, some indication of the pattern of post-war economic boom followed by depression through Reconstruction can be seen.[65]

The drug industry was not merely influenced by the fluctuations in the over-all economy, however, but also by changes in medicine itself. In the decades between 1840 and 1870 regular physicians increased their emphasis on diet and regimen, with particular stress on the use of alcohol as a stimulant.[66] Former practices were not abandoned, but they were used less routinely and, particularly under the influence of such new tenets as homeopathy, smaller doses were administered. There was a major change in attitude from dispensing massive doses of basic medicines to the careful prescription of small quantities of specifically targeted, commercial preparations. Patterns of drug buying changed, with the Civil War marking the turning point in heroic therapeutics[67] and expectations of both physicians and patients changed as a result of the experiences of war and organised, standardised pharmacy service.[68]

MID-CENTURY: DEFINITION

One of the most important factors in the emergence of the modern medical industry in the later nineteenth century was increased precision in the use of drugs, an impetus which came from physicians. There had been great variation of therapeutic practice in the first half of the nineteenth century. The effect of the variety of opinion by pharmacists, small-time pharmaceutical manufacturers, proprietary remedy producers, patent medicine makers, large-scale chemical firms and physicians on medical practices brought confusion. Medical men therefore sought some kind of standardisation of drug prescription and use. Standards for safety and measures of professional status were developed after the Civil War to a new height, particularly through the use of educational criteria, associations and journals. However, pharmacopoeiae became the most explicit standard-setters.[69]

A first attempt to establish a pharmacopoeia in the United States had been made by John Morgan, the founder of the Medical School of the University of Pennsylvania. In 1787 Morgan proposed to the College of Physicians of Philadelphia that a committee be formed to list standard drugs in common use. The committee included physicians from the city but was unable to elicit sufficient support to complete the project.[70] Other attempts were made, but for the most part the Edinburgh or London pharmacopoeiae were used in Philadelphia and elsewhere in the United States.[71] Pharmacopoeiae were needed to standardise drug composition so that the apothecary's compound would bear some similarity to the medicine prescribed. The formulation of a pharmacopoeia by a committee controlled by doctors would further re-establish the primacy of the physician over the pharmacist in therapeutics, since it reduced the possibility of the pharmacist creatively reinterpreting prescriptions.

A variety of pharmacopoeiae had been published in the United States by the middle of the century, including two simultaneously in 1835, when the Philadelphia medical community would not agree to the composition of the committee formed in New York to produce the second edition of *The United States Pharmacopoeia*.[72] The pharmacopoeiae usually included short descriptions of the dosage and use of medicines and sometimes gave therapeutic advice. Although they had no legal standing, pharmacopoeiae were quickly recognised to be of major influence. They were collections of empirical and traditional knowledge and made no attempt to validate the information they provided scientifically. In fact, experiments in pharmacology were rarely made before the middle of the century, except in Britain and France where some work was undertaken by researchers analysing the correlations between chemical constitutions and physiological action.[73]

Whatever the influence of pharmacopoeiae in the period immediately after the Civil War, there continued to be a wide range in the type and quality of drugs sold. The existence of pharmacopoeiae was the only evidence of any trend toward industry-wide standardisation. Even within firms, products varied from batch to batch, without arousing particular concern on the part of producers.[74] The apparent similarity of competing products led, according to one medical man, to an:

> astounding multiplicity of forms and shapes into which different manufacturers are constantly putting articles that ought to possess a standard of unvarying strength and definite composition, so that, busy and hurried as we all are likely to be, the proper doses and standard preparations should be fixed in the mind for instantaneous preparation. . . . Yet each 'house' has its own standard of strength and method of concoction, with no recognized standard to govern the dose or form of preparation.[75]

The growth of pharmacy schools and associations which established professional criteria was another sign of increasing, though also limited, definition within the pharmaceutical community. In 1821 the Philadelphia College of Pharmacy was founded in order to train pharmacists and to provide a focus for the city's community of drug manufacturers by involving them in academic and administrative functions. All the leading manufacturing pharmacists of the city supported the college.[76] After the threat of competition from the Medical School of the University of Pennsylvania, the college responded with a clearly defined academic mission in addition to that of craft training.[77]

The Philadelphia pharmacy community was further held together by a variety of publications. The College of Pharmacy began its journal in 1825. This was the first American pharmaceutical journal and its success led to its reformulation as the *American Journal of Pharmacy* in 1835. It became a nationally respected publication, despite its exclusive ties to the college.[78] Other Philadelphia publications further helped to define the community. One, the *Philadelphia Druggist and Chemist*, was especially successful, appealing even to regular medical men; shortly after its foundation in 1878 it changed its format to include items of particular interest to physicians.[79]

The Philadelphia College of Pharmacy had even greater impact on the pharmaceutical community through its influence in the establishment of other schools and associations which set educational standards before the Civil War. Among them were the Massachusetts College of Pharmacy founded in 1823 (begun as an association, the present school was founded in 1867)[80]; the College of Pharmacy of the City and County of New York, 1829; the Maryland (Baltimore) College of Pharmacy, 1840; and the Chicago College of Pharmacy, 1859. The St Louis College of Pharmacy was founded during the war, in 1864, perhaps with the additional incentive of the army's need for trained medical men.[81] Although this growth was prodigous, even by the end of the century most pharmacists still trained solely through apprenticeship.

The influence of these schools was felt in a number of areas. The Philadelphia College faculty assumed the role of inspector of the drugs on the local market and analysed drugs submitted to them by importers.[82] The schools were instrumental in building the American Pharmaceutical Association (1852) and, by the establishment of their own degrees and of the professional association, they served as gatekeepers.[83] They also pressed for state and federal legislation, and for the enforcement of licensing by local authorities.[84]

The professional image which the degrees and licences helped to create encouraged the establishment of a number of pharmaceutical societies in the United States. These were mostly regional and focused on considerations of problems of business practice and the introduction of new remedies.[85] By the outbreak of the Civil War, drug dealers of every description, from manufacturers and importers to wholesalers and retailers, had developed a sense of common interest. Price fluctuations and the effects of restrictive tariffs had led to extensive speculation about some imported drugs such as quinine.[86] As a response to this, the Philadelphia Drug Exchange was founded in January 1861, just before the outbreak of war. Its main function was to provide a central location for the sale of drugs. This had become necessary because the large number of rural and western merchants now coming to Philadelphia to place orders required a central location for business.[87]

The Drug Exchange soon developed into a trade association effectively controlling competition amongst Philadelphia merchants and displaying an organised, common front to their competitors in New York. No doubt the frequent frauds and generally low reputation of the business influenced the Philadelphia merchants to band together to 'unite for the protection and advancement of their common interests'.[88]

> Differences and misunderstandings in the trade disturbed at times its quietude. Questions of custom and right concerning weight and taxes, discussions as to length of credits to customers, irregularity in prices, attempted frauds upon the fraternity, and a score of other causes, made it desirable that its members should be brought into close and frequent contact.[89]

The establishment of the Exchange was also an effort by the manufacturers, importers and wholesalers to distinguish themselves from druggists in the retail trade. Of course, most members had originally been retailers, but they now felt that the common problems of brokering gave them a separate status.[90] The Exchange did normal daily business, with occasional special meetings of members to discuss legislation or finance. In the post-Civil War period, federal action became a central concern.

Foremost was the lobbying against the stamp tax on medicines, an effort which required the national support of druggists and which met with success in 1884 with Congressional repeal of the law taxing the sales of patent medicines.[91]

Lobbying of Congress was coordinated from Philadelphia with the use of special circulars which the Exchange distributed nationally almost every fortnight from the end of the Civil War until the mid-1870s. These first reported the quantity and type of drugs being imported and methods for merchants to enhance their trade.[92] Whatever the quality of business advice these circulars imparted, it certainly did much to boost the national image of the Philadelphia manufacturers. By the mid-1870s the Exchange had members from New York to California, with over half of the states represented among them.[93]

CONSOLIDATION, 1870-90

By the 1870s the Philadelphia medical manufacturers dominated the region and supplied the bulk of the southern and western markets, regaining their wartime losses. Powers and Weightman, Rosengarten and Sons, Smith Kline, Wyeth and smaller Philadelphia manufacturers all expanded after the war.[94] The post-war boom brought the total number of Philadelphia establishments producing patent or proprietary drugs, pharmaceutical preparations or disinfectants, to 144 by 1882.[95] In that year a census of manufacturers was conducted in Philadelphia which was far more inclusive than the 1880 national census.[96] It found 1581 employees producing $8 114 500-worth of drugs that year. The census also revealed the high income of patent and proprietary medicines; five patent drug manufacturers averaged over $1 100 000 each in the value of their products from workforces averaging only 131. This contrasted, however, with the large number of pharmacists (133) who were producing medicines at the less impressive total value of $2 433 400 and employed 857 people. This still averaged $18 296 per firm, with almost 6.5 employees each.[97]

The difference in the level of income points out the distinction between the large manufacturers of proprietary drugs and the small pharmacists selling a particular specialty preparation for the drug trade while operating a retail business. This distinction diminshed as wholesaling grew, and as 'ethical' pharmaceutical manufacturing took over from pharmacists' production later in the century. It became blurred in the cases of such companies as Smith Kline where most of the products were supplied as raw materia medica and sold either in semi-processed form or fully compounded as brand name products.[98] This combination of both the mixing of compounds, a wholesaler's function, and the processing of raw materials became a new characteristic of the late nineteenth-century drug industry. Since retail drugstores stocked several thousand different items, it became:

> manifestly impractical for a retail druggist to attempt to buy every item in his stock directly from manufacturers. The cost of such a practice would be prohibitive both for retailers and for many manufacturers.[99]

New opportunities for mass distribution presented the pharmaceutical manufacturers with novel marketing problems.[100] Pressures to regularise quality and extend services had been widely felt in other industries. These were first manifested at mid-century in the farm products trade, where commodity dealers sought goods of a more regular quality and quantity, and states began to regulate grain elevators.[101] Then shortly after the Civil War cotton traders formed exchanges to employ brokers to link small farmers and general storekeepers. Their first function was to define and standardise cotton and to arrange for its inspection.[102] Wholesale operations changed significantly after the Civil War for drug merchants, as well as for the related businesses of grocery and hardware. By using the telegraph and relying on railroads, wholesalers could cut the extent of their inventories and operate with the certainty that their orders would be filled on a predictable schedule.[103] By the 1880s when Smith Kline and Company had worked out their quick distribution system, they could usually supply an order within a week.[104]

The new developments in communication lent strength to Philadelphia's drug merchants; but, conversely, they also threatened them. The efficient use of the railways meant that Philadelphia could be seriously challenged as the American medical supply centre. McKesson and Robbins, Schieffelin Brothers and Company, and other large drug wholesalers in New York and Chicago grew rapidly, rivalling the largest of Philadelphia's dry goods and hardware enterprises.[105] Their growth in size and expanded range of products were also facilitated by the use of trade catalogues. Instead of peddling samples in the manner of dry goods salesmen, hardware, grocery and drug merchandisers took bulk orders from catalogues. These were well-structured pamphlets which described products, listed available packaging, and often gave detailed comparisons with other available drugs.[106] Competition through these trade catalogues became fierce as the Philadelphia manufacturers sought to maintain their pre-eminence.[107]

RELATIONS WITH THE MEDICAL COMMUNITY

Despite lucrative financial arrangements between some physicians and pharmacists, there were continued complaints in the second half of the nineteenth century from doctors about pharmacists' activities. In an eloquent plea for physicians to be on their guard against unscrupulous pharmacists, Dr George B. Swayze wrote in Philadelphia's *Medical Times* in 1873:

> In the absence of statistics, I venture the assertion that druggists conduct one-half of the medical practice of the day through the continuous and broadcast dispensation of patent and proprietary medicines, by renewals of physicians' prescriptions, and by other ventures at prescribing for persons over the counter on some general statement of symptoms or complaint by the applicant, either for himself or other members of the family, or for some friend.[108]

Swayze's article was but one contribution to an ongoing debate about the appropriate place for druggists in a medical world in which the physician was supposed to be the only legitimate prescriber of treatment. He blamed the physicians for some negligence, but clearly had no respect for either the skills or the honesty of pharmacists. Swayze did, however, refer to the main argument which pharmacists used to counter such attacks. Pharmacists felt that they could not live by prescription business alone. They argued that they needed to prescribe themselves and to sell patent medicines to stay in business, since the high price of compounded medicines was driving many people to homeopaths, whose treatments were cheaper.[109]

Physicians frequently tried to restrict their relationships with pharmacists. The Philadelphia County Medical Society, the local American Medical Association (AMA) chapter, had been organised in 1849 to provide for the institutionalisation of AMA rules and ethical guidelines. In 1877, an addition was made to the by-laws to deal sternly with the issue of commercial endorsements of drugs:

> Any physician who shall procure a patent for a remedy or for any instrument of surgery, or who sells or is interested in the sale of patent remedies or nostrums, or shall give a certificate in favor of a

patent or proprietary remedy or patented instrument, or who shall enter into agreement to receive pecuniary compensation or patronage for sending prescriptions to any apothecary, shall be disqualified from becoming a member; or if already a member, upon conviction of such an offense in accordance with Article VIII, he shall be *ipso facto* deprived of membership.[110]

A strict line had been drawn between physicians and pharmacists in their commercial enterprises.

Research links between medical men and drug firms, however, were not severed by these rules. Both sides found some links profitable – commercially or scientifically. Gradually, through the last third of the century, clinical tests on drugs began to be made. The Philadelphia physician Horatio C. Wood was one of the first Americans to conduct experiments to establish the clinical effects of various drugs.[111] Wood was Professor of Botany at the University of Pennsylvania from 1866 to 1876 and of therapeutics to 1907.[112] In his pioneer treatise of 1874 on therapeutics he included a standard classification of drugs and a discussion of the effects of small doses of various compounds on man.[113] Wood was also editor of the *Philadelphia Medical Times* in the 1870s and of the *Therapeutic Gazette* in the 1880s. His work is exemplified by his 1885 study of hyoscine (a stimulant alkaloid, like belladonna):

> My attention was attracted by a rather acrimonious controversy in the European medical press concerning hyoscyamine. There was on the market an impure form of hyoscyamine, so called, a blackish liquid. . . . it became apparent that impure hyoscyamine was many times more potent than the pure. I wrote to Merck, asking if he had ever chemically examined the impure hyoscyamine and had obtained anything out of it except hyoscyamine. It appeared that his chemists had isolated an alkaloid which they called hyoscine. This I studied, first thoroughly on dogs, then on myself, then on my wife, then on patients, and published the results; later I received a note from Merck, offering to furnish me without charge any product he had and which I might want for experimentation; also he offered, if I had any chemical research in contemplation, to put all the chemists I needed at my disposal.[114]

The 'acrimonious controversy' in Europe was typical of the disputes over physiological action in the 1880s.[115] By going to 'Merck', that is, Georg Merck, he established contact with a manufacturer which had a worldwide supply network and many scientists working as consultants. Merck was a descendant of the founder of the seventeenth-century Darmstadt pharmaceutical house which had established a New York office in the 1880s. Merck's firm was, even then, one of the world's largest drug makers and its American office became the basis of what is today a major producer, having acquired four Philadelphia firms by the 1950s.[116] Wood maintained his contact with Merck throughout the 1880s and 1890s, but was used less as a staff scientist than as an ornament and occasional consultant.[117]

His activities in research and contact with the industry, as much as his stature in academic medicine, made him an influential man. He served on the board of the *United States Dispensatory* from the 1880s until his death in 1920. Wood used this position to press for greater reliance on drug action as measured in physiology, experimental pharmacology and therapeutics.[118] In recognition of the ability of firms such as Merck to meet high standards, Wood worked towards greater specificity of contents.[119] Collaborations such as Wood's with pharmaceutical firms like Merck were unusual as early as this. Twenty-five years later they would have been even more difficult when the American Society for Pharmacology and Experimental Therapeutics excluded members who worked 'permanently' with any drug makers (though consultancy arrangements were hazy).[120] This action, ironically, encouraged researchers to enter companies directly rather than to try to span different institutional settings.[121]

One of Wood's other aims was to urge the reclassification of drugs in pharmacopoeiae on the basis of physiological action. This paralleled his academic goal of transforming pharmacology into an experimental discipline. Most importantly, he led the way in showing the relevance of particular academic studies to the companies and, conversely, how the industry could assist in research.[122]

Conflict between pharmacists and physicians continued through the century, easing only after drug makers had managed to improve their image. Only then could pharmacists be acknowledged as partners in scientific medicine and not simply as competitors in a cramped market for patients. The growing sophistication of academic pharmacology did nothing to lessen the suspicion between physicians and pharmacists. One commentator wrote in 1881 that:

> As the apothecary advanced from the obscurity of pharmaceutical chaos, and the medical profession reached to him the hand of friendship and professional support, the physician did not foresee

that, through the system of prescription-writing, the sending of patrons to drug-stores for all needed remedies, he would be placing both his professional knowledge and his business interests, day by day, year by year, continuously into the hands of the druggist, and that through these opportunities, the influence and importance of the druggist would so rapidly augment that the said druggist would soon become the formidable business rival of the physician in nearly every practical sense, while the professional consequence and prosperity of the physician *must* proportionally wane.[123]

Despite both passive and rhetorical opposition from physicians, the patent and proprietary medicine trade grew enormously in the 1870s and 1880s, along with the large-scale medicine makers.[124] Physicians themselves paradoxically stimulated some of this growth. By the end of the century proprietary preparations were being routinely prescribed by regular physicians under brand names.[125] Physicians had largely come to accept that the drugs produced by pharmaceutical houses were generally of better quality and more standardised than those prepared by individual pharmacists. Now firmly established, many Philadelphia pharmaceutical companies were well-prepared for the expansion promised by the development of 'scientific medicine'.

3 Company Structure and Scientific Medicine, 1890–95

The 1890s were watershed years for the pharmaceutical industry because of crucial changes in two areas. The first of these shifts came in the structures of the companies themselves, fostered by new opportunities for the exploitation of national markets. Many drug merchants throughout the United States who wholesaled and processed materia medica and patent and proprietary medicines, now grew substantially. In New York, Sterns, Schieffelin, Squibb and Merck imported and produced newly expanded lines of pharmacy products. In the midwest, Parke Davis, Lilly and Upjohn extended their markets,[1] while in Philadelphia, Smith Kline in particular overtook its large competitors, John Wyeth, Powers and Weightman and Rosengarten and Sons, to become the city's pre-eminent drug dealer.[2]

A second crucial change in the 1890s occurred in a few companies, mostly certain small wholesalers, which began to use scientifically and medically trained personnel in a systematic fashion. Such staff became available for the first time as scientific medicine, in particular bacteriology, began to be taught in medical schools.

COMPANY STRUCTURES

Business forms in all sectors of the American economy changed markedly after Reconstruction. As Alfred Chandler points out, American industry established its modern form in this period. Chandler argues that between the 1880s and the First World War, business was altered more by the nation's dynamic economic climate than by public policy, capital markets or entrepreneurial talents. Fundamental changes in processes of production and distribution, 'made possible by the availability of new sources of energy and by the increasing application of scientific knowledge to industrial technology', brought about the modern business enterprise.[3]

Most aspects of Chandler's claim hold as true for the drug makers as for other sectors. However, there are some differences. For example, public policy of various forms did, to some extent, affect areas of the industry. At the end of the century, state and local efforts to manufacture products such as disinfectants, vaccines and antitoxins for public health campaigns competed with some private producers. After 1900 leading manufacturers were increasingly concerned about the quality control of drugs and lobbied the government for laws which helped to rationalise the industry.

Pharmaceutical companies also made use of newly available forms of finance. Larger amounts of capital were obtainable through the developing banks and finance corporations than before. Meanwhile, incorporation laws encouraged the separation of owners from operators,[4] which enabled firms to garner funds through the issue of stocks and shares. Paralleling the pattern of expansion in other industries, drug makers now began to work with the increased security and flexibility allowed by higher levels of fixed capital.

The drug industry in Philadelphia grew almost fourfold in the decade from 1890, an expansion significantly above the national average. By 1900, eighteen establishments in the city accounted for 28 per cent of the national value of drug output.[5] This growth was largely a result of the expanded opportunities afforded by wider sources of supply and more distant markets, which in turn were dependent upon improvements in communications. The Wyeth Company and Smith Kline and French now prided themselves on such remote sources of drugs as the Caribbean, South America and north-western Canada.[6]

With suppliers and distributors increasingly widespread, manufacturers urgently sought coordinating networks. Glen Porter argues that large companies during the 1890s were suddenly faced with a number of new and simultaneous problems.

How could an owner or manager know what was going on in the various locales? How could he make his decisions known to distant employees and see that they were effectively carried out? As the number of different functions performed by a single firm increased, the difficulties grew even more complex. How could the purchasing department supply the right amount and kinds of raw material in the right sequence [?] . . . How could the needs and capacities of the various divisions of the firm be ascertained and coordinated? How could the marketing activities be geared to the rate of production so as to insure a rational flow of goods into the market and thus avoid fluctuations in prices and profits?[7]

At least the problem of distant manufacturing plants rarely faced drug companies: most kept their production at one site and managers usually had close contact with workers.[8] However, those companies which did deal with remote areas, whether as sources for medicines or as markets, now required large ordering and contract operations with the problems that Porter describes. They also needed more efficient warehousing and packaging departments. These were introduced slowly, at first only by the large partnerships like Parke Davis, Smith Kline, and Sharp and Dohme.[9] Then new forms of finance and organisation encouraged family firms to make way for increasingly complicated structures which adapted more easily to large-scale production and expanded markets.[10]

The typical structure of pharmaceutical companies, as with other manufacturing firms, consisted of direct family control over all aspects of production, marketing and sales. Family firms in Philadelphia in 1890 usually had a paternalistic head or a leadership of partners, many of them descendants of the founders. Wyeth and Sons, Powers and Weightman, Rosengarten and Sons, and Smith Kline, all had non-hierarchical structures in which family members controlled major operations using no middle management.[11] In the course of the decade this changed radically with the development of physical departmen-talisation and managerial hierarchies. Professional managers were employed and given charge of separate operations such as purchasing, development and testing, manufacturing, marketing, shipping or sales. In some companies these departments each had administrative hierarchies with parallel structures.[12] Those newly formed companies which grew to considerable size during the last decade of the century were structured from the outset along these lines.[13]

These trends can be seen in most of the Philadelphia companies which survived the decade. By the mid-1890s Smith Kline and French had become Philadelphia's largest wholesale drug house, employing 265 people in 1896.[14] It built its reputation on prompt deliveries, most items being sent out immediately upon receipt of the order. This unique service was stressed in advertisements and trade catalogues, rivalling competitors' claims that 'more than one thousand of our products are [tested and standardised]'[15] or that their drugs were in particularly 'convenient tablets'.[16] Most companies took a week or more to process an order, but Smith Kline:

> could usually have an order shipped within a day, an invaluable service to the pharmacist when he has urgent needs.[17]

A pharmacist or physician, therefore, could expect to receive the goods within a week. The company was able to do this, despite the size and variety of its stock, by rationalising its warehouses and office arrangements and by maintaining a strict hierarchy of specialised clerks. Their shipping department came to look like a large clerical operation with row upon row of desks.[18] Orders were processed on the top floor of the main building and instructions were sent downstairs to the shipping department. Parcels were taken to nearby Reading Railroad Terminal by messenger throughout the day.[19] The firm's reputation for supplying pharmacies and physicians secured stable markets nationally, and many Philadelphia pharmacists regarded it as their principal source of standard goods.[20]

The H. K. Mulford Company was one firm established in the early 1890s which was structured from the beginning with an eye to efficient, large-scale production. The company traced its origins to a prominent Philadelphia drugstore in which Henry Mulford served his apprenticeship while at the Philadelphia College of Pharmacy in the mid-1880s.[21] Mulford became a full partner and then owner within two years of his graduation. He began manufacturing pills in 1889,[22] and his first products were tablets and lozenges, typical of the time, except that they were made with an efficient new tableting machine.[23] Mulford then invited a pharmacy college acquaintance, Milton Campbell, to become a partner and in particular to organise the business aspects of the firm.[24] Campbell was given control over the rate of production which he held in strict coordination with distribution. He then hired a professional manager, A. T. Rickards, who had trained at Godley Commercial College and had worked in the large department store, Strawbridge and Clothier.[25] These appointments assisted the firm to departmentalise into efficient production units earlier than its competitors.

Ethical pharmaceutical manufacturers were not the only drug firms to undertake departmentalisation; even small vaccine farms began to change their structure. For example, when Dr H. M. Alexander expanded his smallpox vaccine business from a small-time cattle farming and medicine-making enterprise into a large-scale production facility, he carefully separated farming from production and shipping. Typical of the many companies started by charismatic entrepreneurs, Alexander kept the sales work for himself.[26]

Prospects were dim for smaller firms which did not develop efficient business techniques. Their sources of finance were unreliable, and their failure rate high, especially among the shoe-string patent medicine makers who often over-extended themselves during brief periods when their products sold well.[27] Among ethical pharmaceutical makers the failure rate seems to have been less dramatic. Existing statistics are inadequate to indicate how risky the business might have been, but most of the large, diversified drug makers survived through this period. Among small vaccine farms, however, the bankruptcy rate was high, particularly after the 1902 Licensing Act dictated that they meet stringent standards. The imposition of such standards forced a third of the firms out of business.[28]

Competition between producers varied in form. Some disputed almost entirely over their local markets while others launched themselves into battles with national rivals. Smith Kline and Company, for example, competed with their Baltimore neighbour, Sharp and Dohme, another wholesaler and processor.[29] Both relied on their wide range of products and their services to pharmacists to maintain huge wholesaling empires.[30] Later in the decade Parke Davis competed fiercely with H. K. Mulford over the title of 'most advanced scientifically'.

The overlap in product lines is striking. All the large wholesalers/ producers offered a full range of standard preparations. In 1895 buyers could choose between Merck, Smith Kline, Parke Davis, Eli Lilly, Sterns, Schieffelin, John Wyeth, Upjohn, Mulford, Sharp and Dohme and many others for a complete line of the basic medicines in convenient forms. For example, belladonna, quinine, arrowroot, and various mercury compounds were all available in a wide range of formulations from each of these companies.[31] Buyers probably based their selection on a firm's salesmanship, or coverage of a particular regional market. The nature of the goods themselves was very similar from company to company.[32] Some buying patterns can be discerned, however. Many of these companies boasted national distribution, though transportation and tradition in fact limited their markets. Ability to develop good links with distant customers therefore became essential for the exploitation of certain markets. An effective organisation and efficient business techniques were the mainstay of such firms.

Firms which expanded through mergers were lauded at the time because of supposed gains from greater efficiency.[33] The tobacco and rollfilm industries became concentrated by 1900 in the hands of two producers.[34] Peter Temin argues that this did not occur in the drug trade because of the nature of technical changes in drug production.

While patents conferred temporary market power on the discoverers of new drugs, many different drugs were discovered and promoted. The existence of numerous patent monopolies worked against the emergence of a dominant firm. The new technology was a method of research rather than a method of production, and that method could not be patented.[35]

Unlike most European countries, the United States allowed medicines to be patented.[36] Few companies, however, took advantage of the law, either because it was an unnecessary procedure when secrecy was a better strategy, or because the poor reputation of 'patent medicines' threatened pharmaceutical manufacturers.[37] Most drugs could be made by a variety of methods and the final products could also be slightly different. This meant that a very large number of patents would have to be taken out on all possible variations of a product in order to protect each marketable item. Such a procedure was not feasible without a large research operation of the type built in the 1920s.[38] Until that time patents were under-used in the drug industry.

However, when we look closely at the industry during this period we do find concentration of a sort,[39] and that concentration was indeed based on science, but not on 'a method of research' as Temin claims. Rather, it centred on a scientific image, a feature which could not be shared equally throughout the industry. Certain manufacturers successfully transformed their image and others did not. While the long-established Parke Davis showed perhaps the most outstandingly successful transformation, most companies which stressed their scientific acumen were founded in the last decade of the century, as in the cases of Mulford and Alexander.[40]

The elaboration in company structure described in this chapter made better use of capital and created a more congenial environment for pharmaceutical research and product development than before. Laboratories could easily fit into large organisations alongside other departments and offices. Extended budgets could be made, allowing development work to be planned for several years ahead.

MEDICAL SCIENCE

The changes in company structure were fortunately timed in the history of the industry. Its close relationship with the medical community meant that as the latter began to adopt medical science, the industry itself had to take increasing notice of the discipline.

In the late 1880s bacteriology was emerging from a long debate over the validity of the germ theory.[41] Though by 1887 at least sixteen disease-causing agents of a bacterial type had been identified, the therapeutic impact of these discoveries had been minimal outside of surgery.[42] Even in surgery, where problems of wound healing had long plagued the profession, resistance to bacterial interpretation was strong.[43] However, by the end of the century, bacteriology had come to be associated with the best of medical science and those institutions which taught and applied it were seen as being at the forefront of medicine.[44] Practitioners began to look to the laboratory for explanations of the cause and spread of disease, and for new means of diagnosis and treatment.

The standard historical explanation for this change in medical practice hinges on the convincing character of particular works by Pasteur, Lister and Koch, and of developments by their followers, especially at the Pasteur Institute and in Berlin, Frankfurt and Munich.[45] That the work of these medical scientists and others such as Roux, Behring, Ehrlich and Kitasato was impressive is certain, but this does not explain how such work came to dominate medical practice. It was the utility of their work which led to its considerable impact. The new generation of laboratory scientists was working not only on theoretical medical science but also on such obviously useful subjects as therapeutics and diagnostics.[46] Their success in producing drugs such as Pasteur's rabies vaccine and practical laboratory techniques for diagnosis gave their work considerable appeal.[47]

Koch's synthesis of techniques allowed bacteria to be selected and differentiated, then grown and tested for pathological effects in a systematic way.[48] He also provided guidelines for the production of pure strains and the identification of types of bacteria by their colony structures.[49] Koch immediately showed the practical value of this work by conducting experiments to pair disinfectants with specific bacteria.[50]

Before the American pharmaceutical companies could attract trained scientists, however, the new studies needed to percolate through their European origins to students in the United States. The main route for the dissemination of these European scientists' work was through medical schools.

Philadelphia's position as an outstanding medical centre played an important part in bringing medical science to the notice of the city's pharmaceutical firms at an early date. The city's medical status was maintained not only by the number of its elite practitioners, but more importantly by its role in training physicians from all over the country. Just as Philadelphia's commerce reached to the west and south, so too its medical schools attracted upwardly mobile students from those regions in particular.[51] The city's medical schools were well-established by the 1890s and anxious to keep abreast of new developments. Since the pharmaceutical industry in Philadelphia was becoming increasingly tied to the medical community, drawing from it both personnel and ideas, companies were soon affected by the new studies.

Koch had few students in the 1880s and the first open classes in bacteriology were given in 1883–84 in Munich and by Fluegge in Goettingen.[52] American physicians and scientists were studying in Germany in great numbers during this period, and it is hardly surprising that two men who were to be influential in establishing laboratory science in the United States studied with early German bacteriologists. William H. Welch, an evangelist for science who was to become a central figure in America's scientific establishment, took courses with Fluegge. When he returned to the United States he was instrumental in the foundation of the Johns Hopkins Medical School, which became the leader in the country for medical sciences. Herman Biggs, who was to establish the bacteriological laboratory of the New York City Public Health Department, took instruction from Johannes Mueller in 1884–85 at the Dental Institute of the University of Berlin.[53]

The number of Americans studying in Germany is not precisely known, but Thomas Bonner has estimated that during the 1880s some 3000 aspiring students and young doctors crossed the ocean to attend lectures from leading scientists and clinicians.[54] Their later significance was more in imparting esteem for scientific research, than the particular learning that they acquired. Some of these scientists then established academic, public health and commercial laboratories on their return to America.[55]

Early bacteriological literature was less vital in the transfer of medical science to the United States, but came to serve as a resource upon which practitioners could later draw. The first journals to publish a significant volume of bacteriological research results were started in the middle of the 1880s. These began with *Baumgarten's Jahresbericht ueber die Fortschnitte in der Lehre von den Pathogenen Mikroorganismen umfassend Bacterien, Pilze und Protozoen* in 1885, and the *Zeitschrift fuer Hygiene* published by Koch's Institut fuer Infektionskrankheiten in 1886.[56] Pasteur's work was gaining renown and in 1888 the *Annales de l'Institut Pasteur* were established and began publishing important work on bacteriology from that institute.[57] Textbooks in English were available from 1886 when Crookshank's *Introduction to Practical Bacteriology* appeared in London.[58] Other English texts appeared in 1887 and 1889, but it was not until 1891 that an American text comparable to Crookshank's was printed, M. V. Ball's *Essentials of Bacteriology*.[59]

Joseph McFarland, a prominent bacteriologist in Philadelphia during the Progressive Era, saw the scientific events of the 1890s as the beginning of an exciting new age for medical research.

[W]hen in 1890 Koch announced the discovery of tuberculin and Behring laid the foundation of the 'Blutserumtherapie', a new era set in, and it was then that representatives of the Federal and State Governments, universities and colleges, hospitals and sanitaria as well as many young graduates just out of their hospital internships, hurried to Germany, took courses, provided themselves with Zeiss microscopes and the newest apparatus, and returned ready and anxious to impart their newly acquired knowledge to others and to add to it as much as possible.[60]

A survey of attitudes towards bacteriology in American medical schools conducted in 1888 largely confirms this sense of promise.[61]

In the 1880s in Philadelphia there were few bacteriologists and only a handful of teaching laboratories where bacteriological work was undertaken. One of the few such laboratories was that at the Medical School of the University of Pennsylvania, which had established a new bacteriological division within the Pathological Laboratory.[62] Between 1890 and 1895, however, teaching and research in bacteriology became increasingly widespread. Henry F. Formad and Allen J. Smith, researchers at the university, published the results of their bacterial taxonomy in the *University Medical Magazine* in 1888 and 1890.[63] Formad, microscopist at the Blockley Hospital, conspicuously supported the germ theory and bacteriology by publishing in the local medical journals, teaching at the University of Pennsylvania and lecturing on news of European scientific medicine after his frequent trips to Germany.[64]

Edward Orem Shakespeare was another prominent local physician who took a strong interest in microbiology, and in 1889 was named the first 'bacteriologist' at Philadelphia General Hospital.[65] Shakespeare had been 'microscopist' and 'pathologist' at the hospital, and his title was probably changed in response to Koch's work. He had recently returned from Germany and Spain where he had studied epidemic diseases, especially cholera.[66]

While the teaching and practice of pathology were hardly synonomous with bacteriological work, by the 1890s many leaders in clinical pathology also taught bacteriology or at least subscribed to the germ theory. For example, at the Medico-Chirurgical College the chair of pathology was given to a proponent of the germ theory, Ernest LaPlace, in 1889. Louis Pasteur specifically recommended LaPlace to William Pancoast, the founder of the college, because LaPlace had been his only American student.[67]

The subject was also taught at the University of Pennsylvania in the regular curriculum from 1889 when Juan (John) Guiteras was appointed Professor of Pathology.[68] According to a student's lecture notes in 1890–91, Guiteras' general pathology course included lectures on the various classes of bacteria, the state of the study of pathogens, and culturing and taxonomical techniques.[69] Joseph McFarland taught an occasional course to third-year students and was given the title 'lecturer in bacteriology' in 1895.[70]

At Jefferson Medical College the first lectures on bacteriology were delivered by W. M. L. Coplin in the late 1880s, and facilities for the preparation of bacteria cultures were established.[71] Jacob DeCosta and D. Brandon Kyle set up a private clinical laboratory at the college in 1893 which was mostly used for diagnostic tests, although some teaching was conducted there as well. Coplin assumed the title of Professor of Pathology and Bacteriology in 1896,[72] by which time bacteriology and clinical pathology were well established in Philadelphia.

In 1892 the University of Pennsylvania constructed a new building to be a Laboratory of Hygiene. The laboratory proved to be an important link between public health workers, researchers and teachers of bacteriology. It also became a critical institution in aiding the nascent scientific work in the local medical industry.[73] It went through two main stages, both of which had significant impact on approaches to medical science in the city.

The first stage was that under its first head, John Shaw Billings, a sanitarian who stressed environmental improvement as fundamental to the prevention of disease. The expressed purposes of Billings' laboratory were to provide up-to-date training in general hygiene and to provide bacteriological and public health instruction for medical students and others. Courses included all aspects of hygiene, including chemistry, engineering and bacteriology. Also to be studied were:

transmissible diseases, prevention, geographical and seasonal distribution and racial susceptibility . . . quarantine . . . disposal of dead . . . domestic and municipal sewage . . . disinfection and sterilization.[74]

Voluntary courses in practical hygiene were offered concurrently for those wishing to have more training for public health work. They included lectures covering ventilation, soil 'from physical and biological standpoints', milk and sewage examination, disinfection and sterilisation.[75] In setting out the programme of the new laboratory, John Shaw Billings commented that:

several so-called hygienic laboratories are simply bacteriological laboratories, the interest in this particular branch of investigation having, for the time being, overshadowed all others.

Our laboratory, however, must provide also the means for chemical investigations of air, water, food, sewage, secretions and excretions, and the products of bacterial growth; for testing the effects of gases, alkaloids, and albumoses of various kinds upon the animal organisms; for investigations in the domain of physics, pertaining to heating, ventilation, house drainage, clothing, soils, drainage, etc.[76]

A. C. Abbott became first assistant, and Albert A. Ghriskey was appointed as assistant in bacteriology.[77] Three early matriculants devoted themselves to bacteriology, all of whom were later to become important in hygiene and public health: Samuel Strayer Kneass (a member of the city Sanitary Committee), Adelaide Ward Peckham and Mazyck Porcher Ravenel.[78] By 1893, twenty-one students were enrolled in the laboratory. Two years later, thirteen of them were concentrating on bacteriology.[79] Billings left in 1896 to be replaced by Abbott, who taught twenty students bacteriology that year.[80]

The laboratory now entered its second stage, with work shifting from environmental intervention to bacteriological analysis. Abbott's work at the institute was very different in orientation from Billings'. He was concerned with the technical capabilities of bacteriology and with teaching a corps of scientific public health workers and researchers, rather than establishing firmer principles for public hygiene.[81]

Before the laboratory had been in operation very long it was discovered that there was a surprisingly small group of men with the peculiar fundamental training that fitted them for the successful pursuit of independent investigations in this important field; and it was discovered that there was and still is but little market, to put it commercially, in this country for men who have been specially and systematically trained in general hygiene.[82]

The techniques and approaches of a new laboratory-oriented medical science were proving themselves in Europe, and American students were carrying them back to the United States. As can be seen from this summary of the Philadelphia schools, they were becoming institutionalised there, too. This was the context to which the pharmaceutical companies now had to adapt themselves.

COMPANY ADAPTATION OF MEDICAL SCIENCE

Medical industry did not immediately begin to produce the drugs which were based on bacteriological theory. Just as their clientele, physicians and pharmacists, were barely coming to terms with such new formulations as the germ theory, so the companies assumed more of the veneer than the substance of scientific medicine.

Besides vague public claims to be scientific,[83] early efforts to include science in a firm's make-up usually focused on laboratories. By the mid-1890s, most of the larger pharmaceutical manufacturers had established some sort of laboratory. Despite their name, these were not centres of investigative science like their European models. Product development was rarely seen as a major function, nor was innovation generally. However, the apparatus and tasks in these company laboratories seemed similar to those in Europe. Test tubes, Bunsen burners, carefully calibrated measures and scales, and acidic and alkali preparations stocked the rooms, and scientists were employed to use them. But the work carried out focused on measurement of existing drugs whose presence in the official or traditional pharmacopoeiae long pre-dated medical science. Drugs were tested to standardise the quantity and quality of their ingredients. Some of this work had been undertaken as early as the 1880s, but it received new impetus from the movement for greater precision embodied in much of scientists' work.[84]

Smith Kline and Company established its 'analytical laboratory' in 1893 when Lyman F. Kebler was instructed to work on the chemistry of drugs.[85] Kebler had been trained in pharmacy at the University of Michigan, in a programme which was institutionally linked with Parke Davis and Company.[86] His familiarity with the latter's practices would have been a highly appreciated asset when he joined its rival, Smith Kline, on earning his degree in 1892. He organised the laboratory the following year, adopting the title of 'Chief Chemist'.[87] The laboratory became specialised almost immediately, concentrating on the analysis of possibly adultered goods which the company bought from suppliers. The company advertised widely that any drugs which did not meet its standards would be sent back.

> It is astonishing how much dishonesty this rule of the firm, as inflexible as the laws of the Medes and Persians, serves to expose – often in quarters from which fraudulent dealing is least expected.[88]

With Smith Kline's expanding trade, investment in the laboratory probably repaid itself quickly in the value of diluted and adulterated drugs exposed as well as the advertising advantages it brought.[89]

By the mid-1890s the functions of the laboratory were expanded. They now included control over some aspects of the actual manufacturing of pharmaceuticals such as elixirs, extracts and tinctures. However, the company still concentrated most of its production in its manufacturing department where relatively simple formulae were mixed in large quantities.[90] As an indication that the analytical laboratory was not initially seen as central to the firm's operation, it was housed in a building three blocks away from the main complex of warehousing and clerical buildings.[91]

Kebler steadily worked to raise the laboratory's status, expanding it from a small testing facility run almost single-handedly to one involving a large staff which contributed regularly to the pharmacological literature.[92] He also increased the importance of his laboratory in an ingenious fashion by cooperating with trained personnel, such as George R. Pancoast, in other departments of the company.[93] Pancoast had joined Smith Kline in 1888 and specialised in their package chemical and essential oil businesses, both of which were very important to the company. Kebler increasingly brought Pancoast and his products into the analytical laboratory, a progression which served a dual purpose. The laboratory found itself handling important products while Pancoast and others started to do research there.[94] Not all pharmaceutical companies had established laboratories, however tenuous, by 1900. Some of the smaller ones had chosen instead to employ one trained scientist to undertake tasks such as standardisation. The Eli Lilly Company apparently tested its drugs even before such a person was employed. In their company history, they claimed that:

As far back as 1884 a company price list declared that '. . . each lot of drug is EXAMINED BY ASSAY before manufacture. We make no extra charge on this account as we consider it our highest duty to *know* our preparations to be of uniform and full strength'.[95]

In the mid-1880s J. K. Lilly, Sr, acknowledged the importance of specialised training by enrolling his son in a two-year course at the Philadelphia College of Pharmacy.[96] Lilly then took advantage of the newly instituted Purdue School of Pharmacy to hire an early graduate, Ernest G. Eberhardt, as a full-time chemist in 1886.[97] Eberhardt undertook spot tests on quality but an incident soon after he arrived convinced Lilly of the need to hire more scientific staff. A customer returned some Extract of Thimbleweed and complained about its quality. Lilly's son sampled the medicine, but it turned out to be poisonous and he was taken severely ill. In response to this mishap his father hired a botanist, Walter H. Evans, who stayed with the company until 1892.[98] He was then replaced by John S. Wright, also from the Purdue School of Pharmacy.[99]

Parke Davis, like Lilly, employed a medical man, Albert B. Lyons, to begin systematic assaying to establish company standards for alkaloidal drugs and their fluid extracts.[100] Even before Lyons was taken on in 1881, a company employee, S. P. Duffield, had published a few articles in the late 1860s in the *American Journal of Pharmacy*. He was not, however, at this stage expected by the company to be a publishing scientist: that was only a minor function and clearly separate from his duties as pharmacist within the company.[101] Lyons began publishing results from his laboratory one year after he joined the company and continued at a productive rate until 1887. He had been a practising MD (University of Michigan, 1868) in the Detroit area when he joined the firm. What the firm's expectations of him were, as a company physician, is not clear, as his medical credentials were not specifically exploited in advertising appeals.[102] He remained with the company long enough to publish twenty-eight articles in five years, before moving to Oahu College in Hawaii in 1888 as professor of chemistry.[103] Lyons's work led to the marketing of 'normal liquids' from the standardised extracts of a number of alkaloidal drugs,[104] and Parke Davis was able to claim that its standardised drugs were more reliable than those marketed by its competitors. The procedures for standardising these early alkaloidal drugs do not seem to have been very expensive. Lyons also published a *Manual of Practical Pharmaceutical Assaying* to guide others who might wish to employ his methods, as well as to advertise Parke Davis' attempts.[105]

A tangential benefit of employing medical men was that they often retained contact with their former schools or fellow students; many also sought academic careers as well as commercial ones. These connections fostered the growing sense of community between the pharmaceutical companies and the regular medical profession, lessening practitioners' suspicions towards their commercial colleagues. The links also encouraged the flow of ideas from academic institutions to the companies, as well as lending the latter a more respectable tone.

While working for Smith Kline and French, for example, Lyman Kebler took advantage of the variety of medical institutions in Philadelphia. Enrolling first as a special student at Jefferson Medical College and later at Temple University Medical School, he studied for an MD between 1898 and 1903.[106] He also maintained close contact with the Philadelphia College of Pharmacy, principally through Professor Charles H. LaWall.[107] Through Kebler's efforts LaWall was periodically employed between 1895 and 1905 as a consulting chemist for Smith Kline and French. The advantages to the company of LaWall's assistance were clear. LaWall himself gained from using the extra facilities in the firm's laboratories, while remaining in his academic position.[108]

Academics may have been more willing to work for companies than previously, but they were also more likely to move out of the commercial sector than before. Thus Lyman Kebler was sufficiently well-qualified by 1903 to consider – and accept – a job from Harvey Wiley as chief of the drug laboratory in the Department of Agriculture's Bureau of Chemistry.[109]

Companies further enhanced their connections with the medical community through the publication of promotional journals. Parke Davis launched two magazines in 1877, *New Preparations* and *The Detroit Lancet* (later changed to *The American Lancet* in 1886 and continued to 1893). *New Preparations* grew into a monthly magazine, *The Therapeutic Gazette* in 1879. The company published *The Medical Age* as a general, semi-monthly from 1883–1906 and *Medicine*, a monthly, from 1895–1907. These were combined into *The Therapeutic Gazette* and became *Therapeutic Notes*. Further publishing ventures were intended more specifically for pharmacists. In 1887 the company started *The Druggists' Bulletin* as 'a monthly epitome of pharmaceutical progress and news',[110] and *Pharmaceutical Notes*. These were later joined together as *Modern Pharmacy*. 'Working Bulletins' began publicising new products and summarising standard technical literature in 1883.[111] The tactic of publishing periodicals based on regular academic journals was followed by a number of producers, most notably the H. K. Mulford Company.[112]

As can be seen, efforts by the companies to associate themselves with a scientific image did not necessarily have much connection with the type of medical science that was being developed in Europe. Some firms undertook botanical expeditions which were out of step in this way. They hearkened back to the type of natural history – or even archaeological – expeditions which had become popular during the century and were associated with the expansion of 'science' in the classical sense. Such expeditions were, nevertheless, associated with the rise of science in the public mind and they served companies well before laboratory-developed drugs became the embodiment of science. The most celebrated of such expeditions were those of Parke Davis, in particular that of Henry H. Rustby to South America in 1885.[113] Adventures of this sort caught the public fancy, often being widely reported in newspapers and leading to popular books.[114] In some ways the American interest in the Amazon corresponded to the British obsession with Egyptology and the Chinese vogue in France during the same period. Besides being useful for public relations purposes, by 1882 Parke Davis was able to introduce forty-six new preparations, mostly as fluid extracts of plants found on botanical expeditions around the United States, British Columbia, Mexico and South America.[115]

For many firms, adaptation to the new ideals of science meant in practice greater standardisation of drugs than before. The touchstones for these producers were the various editions of the United States *Pharmacopoeia* and its supplement, the *National Formulary*.[116] During this period the challenge was to set standards above those of the preceding volume and thereby to appear all the more scientific. Assaying, standardising and 'advanced' nomenclature were the main areas of interest and the easiest ways for these companies to compete along scientific lines. Statements like the following, made at first in the late 1880s, became more and more common during the 1890s:

The United States Pharmacopoeia has omitted to provide for a scientific standard in the determination of the strength of the official fluid extracts. . . . Indeed, as an extra precaution over and above the requirements of the U.S.P., we test all crude drugs by assay wherever practicable. Whatever of discrimination is asked in favor of normal liquids is based solely upon the omission of the Pharmacopoeia to recognize the fact that the only true and scientific test of a fluid extract is the presence of a standard amount of active principle actually ascertained in the finished product, – strength should not alone be determined, as at present, by the quantity of drug employed.[117]

However, standardising, the employment of a scientist, or even the establishment of a small laboratory did not necessarily imply a significant shift in a company's outlook. Thus, for example, despite Lilly's purported interest in science, the company still followed a pattern typical of many drug firms. A major and profitable specialty product which Lilly promoted in the 1890s with the following tale, was a venereal disease remedy:

The story went that McDade, before the Creek Indians were forced westward out of central Alabama, had wangled from one old Negro – who had known another old Negro who had lived with the Creeks – a secret, age-old cure for syphilis, brewed from such components as Smilax sarsparilla (bamboo brier), Stillingia sylvatica (queen's delight), Lappa minor (burdock root), Phytolacca decandra (pokeroot), and Xanthoxylum carolinianaum (prickly ash). Over the years Doc McDade had filtered out various impurities – salt, alum, iron slugs, and assorted nauseating herbs – and now he agreed to ship the necessities for his distillation to Indianapolis. . . .[118]

This story was typical of patent medicine products where an Indian is the origin of the medicine, transmitted to some white man either through the initiation of an entrepreneur or through some other medium, such as the 'old Negro'.[119] It is likely that Lilly made up the formula or bought both it and the story – in the manner of most patent medicine makers. Science played no part in the formulation or promotion of such a remedy.

This example illustrates the ambivalent attitude of most medical manufacturers towards medical science. As a veneer, it was becoming increasingly useful in the promotion of products, but its tenets were not firmly held. Changes in company structure, however, were beginning to encourage a shift from this position as firms tried to adapt to the medical science which was coming to dominate academic institutions. But it was not the private sector in the mid-1890s which undertook the production of the first tangible results of European work: rather, it was the public health bodies. They now became the foremost pharmaceutical manufacturers, using laboratories to produce biological medicines based on immunological theory.

4 Public Health and Diphtheria Antitoxin, 1895–1900

Diphtheria antitoxin was the first biological therapeutic to emerge out of scientific medicine and it dramatically demonstrated the possibilities of a bacteriological understanding of disease.[1] As such it became crucial to the pharmaceutical companies whose area of most dynamic expansion was to be the biologicals. The early days of its production were dominated, however, by public health laboratories. Their involvement in pharmaceutical manufacturing was new, and for a short time eclipsed the more orthodox producers. Their entry into the field stimulated competition with private companies and disputes over many aspects of drug production. Such government activity was challenged as an encroachment on commercial and professional terrain; these demarcations seemed less apparent at the level of operation, however, because of the close scientific and medical links between private and public institutions.

Not only did the public health laboratories initiate production of the biologicals, they also opened up new markets with which commercial manufacturers later dealt. Thus they assisted the companies by demonstrating how the biologicals could be produced – and in many cases they trained personnel who later moved into commerce – and they set into motion a public health campaign which required quantities of medicines which could only be supplied on a commercial scale.

BACTERIOLOGY AND PUBLIC HEALTH

During the decade 1885–95 the number of deaths had been slowly dropping in American cities among a rising population. However, they still seemed unacceptably high. Consumption (or pulmonary tuberculosis), remained the major killer, and childhood diseases seemed to be a growing problem. 'Cholera infantum' (childhood diarrhoea) and diphtheria vied with each other as the major cause of death among children, and trailed only consumption and heart diseases as principal causes over all.[2] Diphtheria had been one of the major causes of morbidity and mortality in Philadelphia throughout the century, usually constituting about 5 per cent of the mortality rate and ranking third among causes of death after infancy.[3]

Diphtheria is a contagious disease which forms a thick membrane over the infected person's throat while simultaneously weakening the victim through high fever and exhaustion.[4] It was commonly confused with other throat conditions although it had been identified earlier in the century as a single, specific disease.[5] Although the disease could be fatal to adults, children were most commonly affected.[6] There were many appalling tales of parents watching their small children slowly die of suffocation from a persistent membrane, or bleeding to death from efforts to clear the throat.[7] Diphtheria lingered in densely populated areas and affected large percentages of the youth in most eastern cities.[8] When the disease was far advanced there was no effective treatment. Cures in the nineteenth century ranged from exorcising demons[9] to various methods of removing the membrane by cutting and tearing.[10] Where it was diagnosed, patients were often put under quarantine, but few hospitals had wards specifically set aside for diphtheria patients until the mid-1890s.[11]

Diphtheria not only appeared to be an endemic disease, it had mysterious fluctuations which could seemingly only be charted, not affected. Some doctors and public health officials were, moreover, becoming concerned with a long-term trend indicating its steadily increasing incidence. Bacteriologists' attack on microorganisms seemed to imply less moral responsibility for disease amongst the general populace while giving public health workers even more active responsibilities. Now it would need to chart the course of disease through bacteriological diagnosing – and ultimately therapeutic and prophylactic intervention. This intrusive form of public health justified both mass vaccination and later the systematic antitoxin treatment. A first priority, though, was the production of diphtheria antitoxin.

THE DEVELOPMENT OF DIPHTHERIA ANTITOXIN

Robert Koch's 1882 isolation of the tubercle bacillus, and the convincing demonstration by Klebs and Loeffler that diphtheria could be definitively diagnosed, lent new significance to laboratory work.[12] Diphtheria became an obvious choice for laboratory research once momentum had developed in the isolation of the causative agents of infectious and contagious diseases. The Koch Institute in Berlin was the centre of such work, as a result of Koch's epoch-making research on tuberculosis and anthrax, and Klebs identified the causative agent in 1883 while Loeffler isolated and cultured it the following year.[13]

Emil Behring and Shibasaburo Kitasato, working at the Koch Institute and funded by the Hoechst chemical company,[14] developed a remedy for diphtheria based on the following procedure: pure toxin, isolated from the Klebs–Loeffler bacillus, was diluted with iodine and injected into an experimental animal in a small dose. The animal, a guinea-pig in the early experiments, was weakened, but as the dose was small it would usually recover. Thereafter progressively larger doses of the toxin were administered until the animal could tolerate doses large enough to kill untreated animals. The guinea-pig had built up an immunity to the toxin, a process which was the subject of extensive speculation. Behring and Kitasato then drained some blood from the animal and let it clot. This separated the red cells from the serum containing the immune products which neutralised the toxin. This serum, they found, could be injected into a second animal so as to create an immunity against diphtheria.[15] Behring and Kitasato published the first notice of their discovery in 1890[16] and by 1894 had extensively tested it at the Charité Hospital in Berlin.[17]

In a series of experiments in the late 1880s and early 1890s, Emile Roux, at the Pasteur Institute in Paris, determined the extent of the toxicity of diphtheria bacilli and showed that a toxin manufactured by the bacteria poisoned experimental animals.[18] In 1894, following the findings of Behring and Kitasato, Roux tried to produce antitoxin in horses in order to manufacture larger quantities than Behring's sheep and guinea-pigs yielded. He rendered several horses immune and conducted clinical tests at Les Enfants Malades Hospital, while watching cases treated in the old ways at L'Hôpital Trousseau.[19] Roux's large-scale production technique proved successful and his results, reported that summer in Budapest at the Eighth International Congress of Hygiene and Demography, created a great stir.[20] By the end of that summer the Pasteur Institute had raised sufficient funds from public subscription to be able to build stables, buy one hundred horses, render them immune, and establish a permanent organisation for the manufacture and free distribution of diphtheria antitoxin.[21]

One distinct difference between the institutional contexts of

Behring's and Roux's work lay in their relationships with commercial interests. While the German scientists were working closely with the Hoechst Company and patenting each development as they proceeded, the French were working in a government-financed institution which had as its long-term goal the widespread distribution of finished products. In France, moreover, the patenting of medicines was prohibited. Behring, on the other hand, set into motion patent applications in Germany, Britain and the United States as soon as clinical trials started. At the Hoechst Company it was common practice for the firm to patent all possible developments in countries where it could, and where such developments might be marketed.[22]

Diphtheria antitoxin was produced in four different institutional contexts. The first experimental antitoxin was made by Behring and tested in Berlin, using guinea-pigs and sheep both as test animals and as serum producers. This earliest work produced only sufficient antitoxin to begin clinical trials, with widespread clinical work seen as somewhat farther off. The second context was that of the first large-scale clinical trials conducted by Roux, using horses as the source of his antitoxin. Roux's aim was the most extensive possible use of the product.[23] When the antitoxin was brought to the United States in the winter of 1894 it was immediately produced for large-scale public health distribution. Not only was this the most feasible institutional context because of the establishment of new laboratories there, it also gave the city and state health departments an active purpose which they were beginning to lack with the decline of environmentalism. The earliest production of the antitoxin in the United States commenced in New York, Washington, Philadelphia, and Boston, but by the end of 1895 public health departments had produced the serum in Buffalo, Rochester (New York), Pittsburgh, St Louis and elsewhere. In addition to German experimental laboratories, the Pasteur Institute and American public health departments, the fourth context was the companies. This will be explored in detail in the next chapter, but the earliest producers, following information-gathering visits to New York, were Parke Davis and Mulford. These contexts implied different scales of production: American public health production began, for example, in large stables well-stocked with inoculated horses and vats of extracted blood and serum.[24]

John J. Kinyoun of the US Marine Hospital Service, along with Herman M. Biggs of the New York Board of Health, were the most influential Americans to bring back European work in bacteriology. Kinyoun's perception of diphtheria antitoxin as something more than the application of bacteriology to medicine was typical of the pioneers of diphtheria antitoxin production in the United States. He immediately saw its commercial significance and thought of massive inoculation as a necessary part of public health work. That the medicine could not be mass-produced at the time, and that there was no sense of appropriate dosage or production standards, did not dissuade him from this point of view.[25] In November 1894 he travelled to Berlin to meet Koch, Ehrlich and Wasserman, witnessed some of Behring's experiments, and sent back information on Behring's method of serum production. When he returned, he added German equipment to his laboratory and began giving instruction on how to produce antitoxin. The Washington laboratory had their first usable antitoxin later that winter, but they were already behind New York in production.[26]

William H. Park made the first diphtheria antitoxin outside Europe in 1894 in the New York city laboratory. He had been appointed chief bacteriologist in 1893 and concentrated on diphtheria diagnosis. Biggs sent instructions directly to him from Europe on methods of preparing the antitoxin which Park implemented immediately. By the time Biggs returned, Park had already produced the serum. So successful was this new attempt that in 1895 the laboratory was divided into a facility for the production of antitoxin and a laboratory for diphtheria and tuberculosis diagnosis. Early in March 1895 Biggs persuaded the state senate to amend the existing laws which would have prevented the commercial production of diphtheria antitoxin. Income from this business was subsequently used to supply the laboratory with equipment, in addition to allowing it to be distributed free throughout New York city.[27]

PRODUCTION IN THE PUBLIC SECTOR

In Philadelphia, the Board of Health accepted a new bacteriological function and decided to appoint someone to concentrate exclusively on bacteriological problems. In 1894 they chose Joseph McFarland (1868–1945) who had earned a medical degree at the University of Pennsylvania where he had studied pathology with William Osler. McFarland had travelled to Germany to work in the laboratories of Julius Arnold and Paul Ernst in Heidelberg and learned bacteriology from Carl Fraenkel at Halle.[28] Upon returning to the United States he was appointed as an assistant to Juan Guiteras in pathological histology and soon became demonstrator of pathological histology and lecturer in bacteriology.[29]

With his European background, McFarland had ambitious bacteriological plans: he aimed to produce sufficient antitoxin for the whole city. He soon became dissatisfied with the city's limited resources in the shared laboratory at the University of Pennsylvania. He therefore exploited his position as a public official and looked for large city-owned stables.

Initially he used stables provided by the Fire Department, but when these proved inadequate, he was given permission to use those of the Police Department, a move simplified by the close ties between the Board of Health and the police. Still dissatisfied with the facilities, and unable to wrest sufficient funds from the city, the Board's work finally lost its appeal for McFarland. In 1895 he moved to the H. K. Mulford Company to begin the commercial production of biologicals, taking his city-gained expertise with him.[30]

In 1896 a special Diphtheria Pavilion had been established at the Municipal Hospital in which antitoxin was administered to promising cases. In their first year they admitted 869 cases, of which 182 died at the hospital, a death rate of 20.9 per cent.[31] The Chief of the Board of Health's division of pathology, bacteriology and disinfection, Dr Alexander Abbott, hoped that this expansion, together with the increase in testing, would encourage City Hall to see the necessity for expanding the production of diphtheria antitoxin. The Mayor's office was willing to see the department produce its own antitoxin, but still refused to fund the operation sufficiently. The city government was particularly concerned that the Board was competing with private enterprise. However, the strategy of restricting its funds proved shortsighted, as, far from undercutting commercial producers by massive production, the Philadelphia Board of Health fell chronically short of antitoxin and was forced to turn to the New York city laboratory to buy from Park. This had become a common procedure for public health departments from around the country and the New York laboratory responded by continually expanding its production.[32]

REACTIONS TO DIPHTHERIA ANTITOXIN

Just as the Philadelphia Board of Health was failing to meet demand for antitoxin, interest in the therapy reached new heights. Diphtheria antitoxin was becoming available in large quantities. Even if tests proved inconclusive and there were problems with the form and concentration of the serum, physicians at least needed to take diphtheria antitoxin into consideration. Medical men were gradually agreeing upon certain results, and it was these that antitoxin producers, whether public health bodies or companies, had to address.

The year 1896 marked an expansion in public awareness of diphtheria and of the possibility of effecting a cure. The *Journal of the American Medical Association*, for example, published six articles on diphtheria antitoxin reporting on experiences of the first full year of use. These papers, presented at state medical society meetings in Illinois, Indiana and Michigan and at the AMA convention held in Atlanta, contained some of the fullest summaries of findings and the most open debate yet presented as to the antitoxin's effectiveness.[33] Some clarification of the results of using antitoxin occurred with improvements in the quality of the serum in the late 1890s. However, problems still occurred with its administration. In 1895 a good batch had 100 units of antitoxin per cubic centimetre, but had been increased fivefold in concentration by the following year. Severe rheumatic pains and other discomfort accompanied the use of this quantity of antitoxin. Concentration of the antitoxin was therefore a major goal for producers because injecting large quantities of anything was risky, or, as one physician put it, 'to inject 10 c.c. of anything into a child is a heroic procedure'. Another prominent physician, Charles T. McClintock, voiced the concerns of those who believed that the antitoxin should be administered in a sequence of small doses, rather than in large ones. The main reason for this was probably the pain it caused, but he had his theoretical reasons too. The disease did not produce toxin all at once, he argued. The antitoxin should therefore be used to stimulate cells to destroy the toxin. This would best be achieved by a sequence of injections to nourish healthy cells.

As can be seen from the general debates over diphtheria antitoxin, interest in the therapy had grown significantly. Commercial companies therefore became increasingly interested in developing a market for biological drugs. Before they could do so, they needed to tackle the present manufacturers of the drugs, the public health bodies. Not only were the public health departments continuing to produce diphtheria antitoxin, they were also threatening to manufacture other medical products, usually tetanus antitoxin, which was made in much the same way as diphtheria antitoxin, and smallpox vaccine, in competition with commercial manufacturers.[34] It became increasingly important for commercial firms to re-establish their pre-eminence in pharmaceutical manufacturing.

Before the companies regained their former positions, however, they needed assistance from the public health boards. As the debate over diphtheria antitoxin also showed, there could be significant problems in its production. The municipal manufacturers had faced these from their first attempts to make the drug. They needed a certain amount of 'know-how', laboratory technique and procedure which was generally undocumented in the first published descriptions of antitoxin production. The first problems encountered by these producers, which had been overcome in Germany by 1890, were associated with the production of the toxin itself.[35] Conditions under which the diphtheria bacillus was cultured had to be maintained with precision, and although the method was relatively straightforward, variables such as acidity had to be closely monitored. Producers also needed to master the tools for the extraction of immunised blood from the horse and techniques for the isolation of blood serum from blood cells on a large scale.

Park was able to overcome these difficulties in his well-appointed laboratory in New York. His experience with diphtheria both clinically and in the laboratory were important in allowing him to develop the necessary techniques.[36] Shortly after he successfully produced the serum he was visited by public health officials from all over the country.[37] Commercial producers followed their lead: among Park's visitors were representatives from two drug companies, H. K. Mulford and Parke Davis. Joseph McFarland learned whatever he could on behalf of Mulford.[38] The companies took advantage of the fact that public health organisations were not, in the end, commercial enterprises and therefore had a duty to advertise their knowledge for the general good. The firms themselves later showed a less charitable spirit.

Having learned what they could from public health bodies, and having lured personnel away from the municipal laboratories, commercial pharmaceutical manufacturers then sought to reduce public production. Two main arguments were used in this campaign: the first was that the municipal facilities were inadequate, and the second that government should not intervene in commercial enterprise by undercutting its market. Firms had one marked advantage in Philadelphia: laboratory facilities in the public health department were poor and staff inadequate. The horses were not sufficiently well cared for and

the stables were decrepit.[39] Although there were no cases of contaminated serum, there was constant concern for sterility.[40] These conditions, as with less suspect conditions in Massachusetts, became the
focus of criticism from commercial producers of antitoxin.[41] Mulford
for example strongly intimated that public health boards were
incapable of maintaining the highest standards and keeping up to date
with the newest procedures.[42]

Together with the steadily-voiced objection to government competing with private businesses, such criticism helped to persuade city
governments to restrict their funding of public health laboratories. So
effective was the campaign that even the New York laboratory was
forced to end its sales of antitoxin by 1904.[43]

The first biological drug, diphtheria antitoxin, emerged in Europe
out of scientific medicine. It was the public health bodies in the United
States, not the commercial companies, who were ready to accept the
challenge of antitoxin production. However, their new role as
pharmaceutical manufacturers was dogged with problems: their
greatest impediment was that they were *not* commercial enterprises,
but dependent upon elected city officials for their funds. These
officials were peculiarly sensitive about infringing on the private
sector, unlike company managements which naturally sought to
expand. Thus, in the public health laboratories' very success lay the
seeds of their decline. Once the commercial firms had learned
techniques from them, they pressed them to relinquish their new role.
The transfer of production from the public to the private sector was
effected by the new mobility of academic, public health and commercial personnel. The medical scientists who led in the public health
production of diphtheria antitoxin now came to lead in that of the
companies.

5 Selling Science: The H. K. Mulford Company

THE MULFORD COMPANY AND DIPHTHERIA ANTITOXIN

The use of diphtheria antitoxin grew enormously from 1895.[1] As more scientists and physicians learned the techniques of production and use, the market for the drug expanded and the number of manufacturers increased.[2] Public health departments provided both the major market and the training ground for antitoxin production.[3] The two major commerical producers of the antitoxin, H. K. Mulford and Parke Davis, both relied on the experience gained from the pioneering work of the New York public health laboratories.[4] And both sought to regain private control of the production of biologicals. The use of science was beginning to have very tangible results in the private sector.

The story of this development was epitomised in the case of the H. K. Mulford Company. The Mulford Company began as a small manufacturing pharmacy, employing twelve people at incorporation in 1891, with a local clientele yielding $35 000 in the first year.[5] By the early 1890s Mulford had already acquired a reputation for high-quality products. The firm specialised in lozenges, elixirs, antiseptics, liquors, tinctures, syrups and fluid extracts – much the same range of preparations as their Philadelphia competitors.[6] Their successful start made it possible for them to expand from their Eighteenth and Market Street offices to 2132 Market Street in 1893 where they erected their efficient tableting machines and produced a large selection of standard and original preparations.[7] The 'machine for manufacturing compressed pills', patented by H. K. Mulford with co-inventor Oberlin Smith,[8] was credited by company employees for changing 'the character of the business from that of a retail drugstore to the greater business of a manufacturing establishment' and bringing 'extraordi-

57

nary popularity' to the firm.[9] These machines produced soluble tablets in contrast to the insoluble pills and disagreeable powders sold by most other firms. Mulford's reputation, confirmed in an editorial in *Practical Therapeutics*,[10] rested on the ability of its tablets to disintegrate in water, in contrast to those which 'pass through the entire intestinal tract and are expelled practically unchanged'.[11]

Before the production of biologicals, the company relied on its line of common remedies. Then as today, the best-selling medicines were for relief of dyspepsia, headache, sore throat, constipation, cough and anaemia. The company also sold popular tonics, antipyretics, antiseptics, and even an aphrodisiac.[12] A remedy for colds was offered which contained small quantities of some of the most common of the heroic therapeutic agents from earlier in the century: strychnine, morphine, quinine, and arsenous acid;[13] a specific for chlorosis, or 'female anemia', was available, chocolate-coated if desired.[14] By 1893 the company was offering over 500 individual items[15] and about five times that number only seven years later.[16]

Mulford's strategy of exploiting its tableting machines to produce the largest possible range of drugs was devised by Milton Campbell, president and part owner of the company.[17] By 1893 Campbell had elevated himself above the routine aspects of drug production and distribution and was able to take a longer-term look at the development of the industry. Campbell's position as a company manager rather than a manufacturing pharmacist encouraged him to take this approach. An initial step in his programme for developing the company was to establish branch offices. The first of these, the Chicago depot, was opened in 1893 'for the better accommodation of our Western patrons'.[18] From an early strategy Campbell's plan blossomed into a worldwide network with offices in Toronto (1900), Mexico City (1911), and fifteen other American cities. By the First World War, Mulford had branches in Honolulu, Buenos Aires, Wellington and Auckland, New Zealand and Durban, South Africa.[19]

Milton Campbell's next plan had even more far-reaching results for the company: he initiated the production of diphtheria antitoxin. In early November 1894 he hired Joseph McFarland from the Philadelphia Board of Health and his work in the Police Department stables, and installed him in newly built stables bought especially for him in Fairmont Park. At the 'Biological Laboratory' McFarland was given almost free rein to develop a marketable diphtheria antitoxin along the lines of his Board of Health procedures.[20] In addition, he was able to collect snakes with which to begin antivenom research.[21] This and other work in toxicology was seen as potentially, if not immediately, commercially feasible.[22] The employment of McFarland was the first direct effort on Campbell's part to enact a policy of active product development through laboratory science. Campbell realised that the quickest way to acquire the expertise needed to produce diphtheria antitoxin would be to hire someone who had worked in a public health department which had already manufactured it. Like most physicians and PhD scientists to follow McFarland, he was brought into the company on a part-time basis. Meanwhile he was able to continue lecturing in bacteriology at the Medico-Chirurgical College and to maintain a small private practice. He was given a good salary (more it seems than the $3000 he earned working part-time at the Board of Health) and his own skilled staff.[23] Implicit in Campbell's offer was the possibility that if things went well McFarland could direct a growing division of the company for the manufacture of biologicals and into which a substantial amount of research would be carried out.[24]

Both Henry Mulford and Campbell had followed the early reports of antitoxin production.[25] The first report of antitoxin use in the United States, of Louis Fischer's trial in New York published in the *Medical Record* of 6 October 1894, was noted in a running bibliography kept at the company.[26] McFarland was probably known to them and already an attractive proposition. An ambitious man in his early thirties, McFarland was conspicuous in his positions at the Medico-Chirurgical College and the Board of Health.[27] He had studied bacteriology in Europe and was regarded as a promising young man in an expanding field. Furthermore, he was probably frustrated with the unsettled politics of Philadelphia public health and its half-hearted commitment to bacteriology. There is no evidence of any hesitation on his part when Campbell tendered his offer.[28] For the company, the investment was hardly a great risk. Apart from McFarland's salary, the only expenses were for the stable, a few horses and a minimum of laboratory equipment. The company's profits were high,[29] McFarland seemed available, and Campbell made a quick decision to attempt the production of biological drugs.

A parallel development took place in Detroit at Parke Davis. In February 1895 the firm hired E. M. Houghton from the University of Michigan where he had worked on the standardisation of botanical drugs. Houghton was appointed Junior Director under Charles McClintock in the newly established Medical Research and Biological Laboratories.[30] The three-month difference in commencement was insignificant: the two companies operated on an equal footing for the first few years of the American production of antitoxin. It was, however, a bone of contention between the companies, as each claimed to be the first to conduct organised scientific research and the first to manufacture antitoxin.[31]

Diphtheria antitoxin was produced within a week of McFarland's arrival at Mulford's Eaglesfield Street laboratory.[32] The company gave him good laboratory facilities and allowed him to employ first a stable-hand and then a scientific associate, Professor Leonard Pearson of the University of Pennsylvania's Veterinary School.[33] Pearson had studied in Germany, spending some time in Koch's laboratory learning bacteriology. Thus, besides being a veterinarian, he was a member of the elite medical science fraternity which had formed its academic attitudes in German universities.[34] Pearson's early involvement with the company was also one in a series of links between Mulford and the University of Pennsylvania which were instrumental in helping the firm make the move from a typical producer of high-quality medicines to a leading developer of new products. Within a few months McFarland had brought in other part-time staff from the university. John Adams, professor of surgery in the Veterinary School and the assistant demonstrator of pathological histology, McFarland's colleague at the Medico-Chirurgical College, both soon became affiliated with the company.[35] An early advertisement promoted this staff:

> The Biological Laboratory . . . is thoroughly equipped for original research and the preparation of the various biological products. It is under the personal direction of Joseph McFarland, M.D., Professor of Pathology and Bacteriology, Medico-Chirurgical College, assisted by C. W. Lincoln, M. D., Assistant Demonstrator of Pathological Histology, University of Pennsylvania. The horses are under the direct supervision of J. W. Adams, V.M.D., Professor of Veterinary Surgery and Obstetrics, University of Pennsylvania.[36]

Mulford's first antitoxin was produced in November 1894, at the same time that the Philadelphia Board of Health was forced by its own low yield to place its first order of $90 worth from Behring.[37] By the spring of 1895 the biological laboratories were able to begin marketing the first batches of diphtheria antitoxin, but had not yet been able to gather the equipment needed to test them.[38] McFarland took advantage of his earlier connection (through the Board of Health) with the Laboratory of Hygiene at the University of Pennsylvania to test his first batch of antitoxin there. Henry Mulford also had ties with the university.[39] He counted as a friend the influential chemist and later Dean, Edgar Fahs Smith, and also drew upon the help of Alexander Abbott, David Bergey and George M. Meeker, Dean of the Post-graduate School of Medicine.[40] With such contacts it was not difficult to arrange for testing at the university. Mulford made a virtue out of its lack of equipment and advertised that:

> each lot of the Mulford Diphtheria Antitoxin was submitted to confirmatory tests by the Department of Hygiene of the University of Pennsylvania, thus early placing the testing of antitoxin beyond commercial control.[41]

Collaboration with the laboratory at the university lasted almost two years, after which the company felt that it was advantageous to do its own testing as part of its laboratory expansion and to have total control over this sensitive area, which could no longer be left 'beyond commercial control'. In the interim, the collaboration seems not to have been questioned at the university and no special arrangements were made to account for the difference between occasional diagnostic tests of pathological materials and a continuing product-testing operation.[42]

In little over a year Mulford had sold 40 000 doses of antitoxin and was building a major advertising campaign around favourable reports from physicians and public health departments which routinely employed the product.[43] There was one particular difficulty in selling diphtheria antitoxin: overcoming widespread resistance to it. The most significant problem was that created by the difference between serum therapy and all other known therapeutic methods. For many practitioners, the conceptual change seemed impossible to grasp. Some groups, however, adopted an amalgam of their own points of view with that of the bacteriologists. For example, the technique could be seen as a kind of combination of homeopathic method and humoral theory.[44] Antitoxin was derived from a product, the bacterial toxin, which would induce the disease, just as homeopathic medicines were derived from products which induced symptoms similar to those of the disease being treated. The toxin was then diluted in the bloodstream of a horse, as homeopathic drugs were diluted by repeated fractioning. Some homeopathic physicians therefore accepted serum treatment while continuing to disregard most other aspects of the scientific medicine of the time.[45] The use of diphtheria antitoxin also appealed to those who clung to humoral explanations because an injection of antitoxin seemed to act by balancing the toxic state of the blood.

Although these conceptualisations of the operation of the medicine at least favoured its use, scientists argued that they had to be supplemented by an educational campaign which explained exactly how the drug fitted into bacteriological theory.[46]

The initial success of Mulford's diphtheria antitoxin encouraged the company to expand the laboratory's functions, including that of education. The laboratory was now expected to perform three main tasks: the development of new biologicals, the improvement of techniques for standardisation, and the presentation of an image of the company as an enlightened, scientifically sophisticated firm. Tetanus antitoxin, which had been announced by Behring and Kitasato along with diphtheria antitoxin,[47] was the second biological drug produced.[48] The feeling at the company was that 'all disease would soon be conquered by anti-toxins'.[49]

> It seemed so easy. All that need be done was to grow the germs in quantities, filter off the toxin, inject it into horses in increasing quantities until the antitoxin was good and strong, draw off some of the horse's blood, let it clot, inject the serum into a human patient and he was safe.[50]

The laboratory staff tried this straightforward technique on almost all known diseases.[51] This research programme was met with frustration and failure because few other bacteria gave off appropriate toxins.[52] Despite the eventual failure of this approach, other biological remedies were quickly developed using similar techniques.[53] By 1898 eleven types of products were being manufactured in Mulford's biological laboratory, including antimeningitis, antistreptococcus, antidysenteric and antipneumonococcus sera, as well as rabies vaccine (Pasteur method), and anthrax vaccine.[54]

The standardisation of diphtheria antitoxin and other products was perhaps particularly frustrating. Behring had devised a rough method for assessing the toxicity of diphtheria serum by measuring the time it took for a guinea-pig to die after being given a specified dose. This quantity was termed the 'minimum lethal dose' (MLD) and the antitoxin was measured in terms of the quantity needed to neutralise, for example, 10 MLD.[55] This method was extremely cumbersome and Behring, Ehrlich and other bacteriologists, as well as commercial and government laboratories, were all working to improve the technique. Ehrlich in fact arrived at a suitable solution in 1897 which was quickly adopted by McFarland and later by the United States Hygienic Laboratory for industry-wide standardisation.[56]

The procedure for standardising antitoxin with a neutralising toxin served the additional function of answering critics who suspected the medicine of operating as an internal antiseptic, killing bacteria rather than counteracting their products.[57] Antiseptics were added to preserve antitoxin, at first carbolic acid and later a less toxic preparation, trikresol, but the company asserted that:

> the theory advanced by those opposed to serum therapy, that antitoxin may derive its therapeutic value from the presence of the antiseptic contained therein, is a fallacy and without foundation.[58]

Apart from answering critics with the weight of a good laboratory behind him, Campbell recognised the competitive advantage of standardisation in the appeal it held for physicians.[59] Mulford quickly became a leader, together with Parke Davis, in standardising its wares and by 1897 had an extensive analytical laboratory concentrating on this problem.[60]

The most successful function of the laboratory was its third charge, the enhancement of the company's scientific image. In the crudest terms, it was stated explicitly in advertisements that Mulford 'is universally conceded to be the most complete and scientific [company] in existence. It embodies the latest development of science';[61] so effective was this promotion that it was even echoed by the *Philadelphia Medical Times*:

> Manufacturers of this character deserve unstinted commendation as public benefactors. The laboratories of the H. K. Mulford Company are, in point of scientific equipment, the most complete in existence, and are under the immediate personal control of eminent scientists.[62]

The achievement of this reputation by the late 1890s was an end explicitly sought by Milton Campbell and Henry Mulford. Influenced by his training at the Philadelphia College of Pharmacy, Campbell in particular wished to stress that pharmacy was a professional activity, a branch of medical science.[63] Campbell even held that pharmacists should take the Hippocratic oath 'to serve the public and the profession altruistically'.[64] As a result of this tenet, Campbell claimed that he intended 'to develop the ideals of medical practice' at the company, as he explained in a later interview:

> The term 'develop' is used advisedly for at the time the H. K. Mulford Company was organized as a corporation there were no

laws obliging the pharmacist or the manufacturing house dealing with the materia medica to adopt the standards of the United States Pharmacopoeia, consequently, the condition of the drug market was such as to make it very difficult to carry out the rules of medical ethics in a practical manner.[65]

He felt that a commitment to science dictated that:

the members of the profession are . . . under obligation to donate the results of their observations and experiences to the common fund of knowledge created by the medical profession and known as medical science, receiving in exchange therefor the results of the knowledge and experience of the entire profession.[66]

Campbell contrasted this to the normal practices of the industry, which was ruled by the 'commercial ideal of competition', according to which most manufacturers, even producers of ethical pharmaceuticals, tried to keep the composition and methods of manufacturing secret. He thought that his company could go beyond the crass 'creation of a demand by the usual commercial methods of advertising'.[67] and saw his form of advertising in a completely different light.

In many ways Mulford's approach to advertising was unique. For Campbell the projection of an image of the company as science-based was of paramount importance. This was enshrined by 1900 in a code of practice, a 'Statement of the Relations of the H. K. Mulford Company to the Medical and Pharmaceutical Professions'.[68] The statement included a number of points, occasionally changed to adapt to company policy,[69] but which placed the company in a unique position with regard to commercial or medical ethics. The first point was perhaps the most crucial in distinguishing the firm from patent medicine makers since it promised to eliminate 'monopoly obtained either by secret formulas or processes or product patents.'[70] The second part of this pledge was dropped by 1912 when the company began to patent a number of items.[71] It also pledged itself to scientific integrity and open publishing, laboratories for standardisation, testing and research, and to accuracy in advertising. The company claimed that they were contributing not only to the reputation of the profession, but also to the discovery of new therapeutic agents.[72] However unusual this approach was at the time, it was an effective means of promotion. The company encouraged potential buyers to believe that it was objective and therefore to be depended upon for reliable scientific therapies.

EXPANSION: THE MOVE TO GLENOLDEN

As soon as antitoxin production was well established, McFarland needed to expand from Mulford's city stables to a site where a horse farm and new laboratory buildings could be constructed. In 1896 a suitable location was purchased eight miles south-west of Philadelphia in Glenolden, Delaware County. The facility, the pride of the company for forty years,[73] had large stables, separate laboratories for biological research and veterinary practice, and a glasshouse and instrument shed. The main building complex covered forty acres with 160 acres of prime farmland nearby.[74] In addition to the horses used in antitoxin production, a herd of cattle was kept for vaccines and a building was erected for vaccine production.[75] The Glenolden plant was described as being 'in an agricultural country particularly noted for its healthful surroundings and beautiful rustic scenery'.[76] It had also that perfect balance necessary for business and farming:

> The farms are entirely removed from the city influences, but are within easy access of our executive offices. Railroad and trolley communication enable us to fill orders from the fresh stock in our laboratories at very short notice.[77]

The vaccine laboratories and the rest of the layout were designed 'after careful inspection of the leading vaccine establishments in Europe and America', and the construction was effected 'in the most complete and scientific manner'.[78]

> The buildings embody all the latest features of sanitary engineering with the details observed in the construction of modern hospitals and hygienic laboratories.[79]

Construction materials were of 'stone, cement, metal, slate, and porcelain-finish'[80] for ease of disinfection, and water sources were carefully guarded from contamination.[81] The most scrupulous sanitary standards were to be followed for veterinary surgery, and the preparation and packaging of remedies.

Glenolden was one of four antitoxin farms which were visited by the Pennsylvania State Board of Health in 1896 when it assessed potential suppliers.[82] The others were in Chicago, Detroit (Parke Davis) and Washington, DC (National Vaccine Establishment). Mulford received by far the best report from the commission, not surprisingly since it was the only local firm and one of the state inspectors was John W. Adams, a Mulford employee.[83] There were three main criteria for the

assessment: the health of the animals, general sanitary conditions –
especially the procedures for injecting animals, the extraction of blood
and the separation and packaging of serum – and the presence of
trained personnel.[84] Besides the advantages just mentioned, Mulford
rated highly because it had been able to provide new stables and had
hired McFarland and his support staff. In later years the farm
continued to recieve glowing reports from public health departments
in north-eastern states, and was favourably assessed after 1902 when
the US Hygienic Laboratory took over systematic inspection.[85]

The problems in scaling up production at Glenolden from the
laboratory level to large batches were quickly overcome. For diphtheria antitoxin this meant that blood had to be collected from
immunised horses and allowed to clot. It was then suspended in
cheesecloth over a collecting vessel into which the serum would drip.[86]
Horses yielded 'considerable quantities' (two or three litres)[87] of blood
which would be immediately transferred to the 'blood room'[88] where
the antiseptic would be added. Glenolden was designed with its
laboratories and stables adjacent to promote efficiency.

Unskilled laboratory tasks and packaging were performed by
women. Photographs of even the earliest production laboratories
show rows of white-coated, hair-netted women preparing syringes,
sealing glass tubes and sterilising vials.[89] 'The girls' were the objects of
attention of visiting pharmacy students[90] and formed separate social
groups.[91] Though some stayed for many years, none was ever
promoted above routine tasks or to overseeing other women.[92] They
were, however, viewed with respect, especially since they performed a
very useful function. Referring to those who filled tubes with
glycerinised lymph for smallpox vaccination, the company claimed:

> The system of division of labor adopted by us, in which one
> individual executes but one kind of work, enables our employees to
> achieve the skill of specialised workers; consequently each step in
> the preparation of our virus is directly controlled by a skilled
> employee.[93]

Women's uniforms and men's white coats were provided by the
company and sterilised daily[94] and their work stations washed as
frequently.

While the women stayed indoors undertaking delicate tasks, young
boys helped as stable-hands and black labourers worked in the fields.[95]
Unlike companies such as Smith Kline where employees could work
their way through the manufacturing department into middle-level

management, at Mulford there was little employee mobility in the first twenty years. Scientific endeavours seemed to require scientifically specialised tasks.

As the company expanded, an increasing number of trained people were employed. Between 1896 and 1911 separate laboratories were built for each of the eleven types of products, cold storage facilities were added to hold stocks of vaccines in case of emergency demand, and the main offices moved three times within downtown Philadelphia.[96] After 1900 the number of items offered stabilised at around 2500 and the scientific staff exceeded thirty.[97] By 1910 the company had 950 employees and grossed approximately $3 million.[98]

EDUCATING THE MARKET

The crucial task in assuring that diphtheria antitoxin and the other biologicals being produced at Glenolden were actually used, was to educate potential users. The basic message was clear:

Don't be afraid to use antitoxin.
Don't be afraid of a large dose.
Don't wait for result of a culture before use.[99]

Antitoxin had not only to be portrayed as an effective cure statistically and epidemiologically, it also had to be seen as a benevolent therapy, easy to use and comprehensible to the average physician.

Great effort was made to 'place in the hands of physicians and pharmacists . . . scientific information concerning [new drugs] just as soon as sufficient data were published by medical scientists. . . .'[100] This was part of 'an educational propaganda':

in which booklets, pamphlets, stock-lectures, lantern slides and moving pictures were employed, all of such a scientific character that universities and boards of health freely used them for educational purposes.[101]

Although direct contact with persuasive salesmen was the best means of imparting information, pamphlets were the most common source of information. The style of publications changed over the years, remaining 'serious' and 'scientific' in appearance but variously taking the form of sales leaflets, general information pamphlets, scientific reports (either reprinted from a journal or mimicking scholarly form), or even the style of review articles, summarising the literature and debate over a therapy. Their content varied far less. Generally the drug would be introduced first, rather than the company, which was sometimes identified on the title page only as the pamphlet's publisher. A discussion of the therapy would follow. Explicit instructions would be given for dosage, administration and follow-through, with careful distinctions made for differing forms of the illness. Early pamphlets (from 1895 to 1898) placed these instructions within the context of basic bacteriology and immunology, explaining the relationship between bacteria and toxin and the neutralising effect of antitoxin. For diphtheria antitoxin, Mulford's product was presented by means of a description, with photographs, of how the product was made. Much was made of the Glenolden plant, the sterile laboratories and testing facilities. Laboratory heads were named, complete with academic and hospital affiliations, discreetly followed by a list of Mulford's biological products, confined to one page and in small print. Prices were usually not included but could be found in separate catalogues or price sheets.

A favourite selling device was to advertise the epidemiology of diphtheria with the statistical effect of antitoxin. This was presented in one early pamphlet by quoting the mortality rates from some unspecified place: deaths ranged from 34.8 per cent to 62.5 per cent without antitoxin, but from 4.6 per cent to 17.64 per cent with the drug.[102] Later pamphlets showed full epidemiological charts. An advertisement from 1905, for example, showed the mortality rate for diphtheria from 1893 to 1904 for Baltimore, Newark, New York, Philadelphia and Rochester (New York) with impressive reductions following the use of antitoxin after 1895.[103]

Another advertising technique consisted of providing the reader with reusable information. Some price lists contained 'A Condensed Glossary of Biological Terms' or a guide to common diseases and frequently used remedies.[104] One pamphlet offered eight colour plates of bacilli charts, as an aid to identification.[105] Others had extensive scholarly bibliographies, diagnostic charts or summaries which might be useful in preparing lectures. In 1916, for example, Mulford offered a wall chart showing the official changes in the ninth revision of the *US Pharmacopoeia*. The message was not left to the dispenser's imagination:

NOTE – Mulford Pharmaceutical and Biological Products conform to the Standards of the New Pharmacopoeia and in many cases Conform to Standards which are Considerably More Stringent than those of the U.S.P.IX. The Mulford Label is a Guarantee of Purity, Accuracy and Reliability.[106]

By 1900 Mulford had supplemented its occasional pamphlets with an organised series of 'Working Bulletins'. The first of the bulletins, 'A Treatise on Bacterins (Bacterial Vaccines); Theories of Immunity, and of Bacteria Therapy; From a practical standpoint and intended for the general practitioner', went through at least six editions. The Bulletins were typically more than fifty pages in length and included a complete review of the literature relevant to a particular product. They presupposed only a limited familiarity with bacteriology terminology and techniques and no knowledge of the specialised medical literature. By 1917, twenty bulletins were available on request, in addition to eight 'informative' (as opposed to advertising) brochures.

In June 1912 the first number of yet another form of promotional literature was published by the company, the *Mulford Digest*.[107] Edited in a separate downtown office by Dr George M. Gould, this periodical assumed the style of a mainstream medical journal. It had a board of editors and its layout, print and binding was much like the *Medical Record*. Subtitled, 'Devoted Particularly to Serum-Therapy, Bacterin-Therapy, Vaccine-Therapy, Immunization, and Drug Standardization', the quarterly published a potpourri of laboratory and clinical reports, reprints from textbooks, reports from the company laboratories and sections of informational pamphlets. Some of what the *Digest* printed had been published by company workers in other journals,[108] while other papers were otherwise unpublished addresses and lectures.[109] The *Digest* was also used as an authoritative source in other Mulford advertising, as when the recommended dosages for Typho-Bacterin were given in the *Mulford Working Bulletin* on typhoid.[110]

Mulford salesman were trained to present scientific information in great detail. They were aided in this by collections of photographs and a series of lantern slides illustrating the diagnosis of diphtheria and tetanus, Mulford's method of producing antitoxin, and the different packages available. This method of direct education reached a peak after the war with the opening of the Mulford School of Bacteriology and Immunology. Intended primarily for company employees, the lectures were open to local physicians who wished to attend at no cost. Twenty-five Mulford workers were paid full salaries while attending classes. Dr Frank M. Huntoon, formerly professor of bacteriology at Cornell University, offered three consecutive courses in 1919. The first, on general bacteriology, included instruction in sterilisation, culture techniques and microscopy. This was followed by an advanced course covering pathogenic organisms, prophylactic action and therapeutic use of biological products. The course was attended primarily by the sales staff of the company, the material being too elementary for trained scientific workers.[111]

In advertising to pharmacists, Mulford stressed that its products would draw more general business. One pharmacist testified in 1900 that:

> MULFORD'S ANTITOXIN is the biggest hit I ever made in the way of advertisement with physicians. I do not know of a single preparation like it; the fact of having Antitoxin (Mulford's) in stock is worth a $25.00 advertisement to any store that is trying to sell to physicians.[112]

Mulford went further than their competitors in becoming associated with the most advanced medicines, but they never quite ruled the market. Parke Davis took equal trouble to stress the quality of their standardised fluid extracts, using reference to Houghton's laboratory in much the same way that Mulford made use of McFarland's.[113] They also stressed their longer record of drug standardisation. 'For twenty years before the United States Pharmacopoeia of 1890 gave it half-treated recognition', they had applied chemical standardisation.[114] Parke Davis was a formidable rival. Their scientific reputation grew rapidly as they hired more University of Michigan graduates and adopted strategies similar to Mulford's for the enhancement of their corporate image. Both companies had vociferous supporters and extensive sales. Edwin Rosenthal, a prominent Philadelphia physician and friend of Joseph McFarland, gave a tempered summary of the reputations of competing companies and public health departments in 1896.

> Antitoxin . . . is in the hands of the large manufacturing establishments, which, by reason of unusual enterprise, greater capital, wider scope and standard methods, are enabled to produce standard and stable articles. . . . Its manufacture should be placed in the hands of the most competent.[115]

Since antitoxin was not proprietary, Rosenthal continued, 'its virtues and reputation depend more upon the honor and reputation of those who manufacture it than upon its name'.[116] After describing the Hoechst, Schering and Pasteur Institute serum, Rosenthal recommended the Mulford product. The New York City Board of Health product was 'of value' and that of Philadelphia had 'utility'. Others, however, should 'be questioned'.[117]

Mulford could not keep ahead of its competitors for long. By 1905 other producers of biologicals were perfecting methods similar to those used by Parke Davis and Mulford. Competition with public health departments also grew sharper during and after 1896. In addition to the large-scale production of antitoxin in New York, Massachusetts was making enough to satisfy that state's needs and many public health departments, like Philadelphia's, were producing much, if not all of what they needed for their own use.[118] By 1900 the inroads this production made on commercial markets were threatened by the common practice in most states of making antitoxin available free of charge to physicians who treated needy patients in dissemination programmes modelled after those of New York and Philadelphia.[119] Mulford brought suit a number of times to try to persuade state legislatures to curtail this 'interference with private enterprise' but failed in Massachusetts because they could not present convincing evidence that the denial of that particular market cut significantly into their profit.[120]

In 1904, however, an injunction against the public health department in New York city succeeded in stopping the widespread sale of their antitoxin.[121] That injunction lasted only two years because Park's customers in other public health departments insisted on continuing to purchase his preparation, having achieved good results from it over a number of years.[122] Mulford's only response was to provide special prices for public health departments, a procedure which cut substantially into the company's profits.[123]

RELATIONSHIP WITH THE MEDICAL COMMUNITY

Mulford maintained excellent contact with the mainstream of the medical community. This was necessary both to assure close ties to its market and to enable it to draw from clinical and scientific experience. Hospital trials for its products were particularly useful and the company advertised its 'extensive connections with hospitals'.[124] Bacterins, for example, were tested at Bellevue and the New York Hospitals.[125] Outside consultants to the firm who also held hospital appointments were prized by the company, as was the case with G. M. Dorrance, who tested an experimental cancer 'vaccination' at St

Agnes' Hospital, Philadelphia.[126] Ferri Compound, an antimalarial drug and a 'most popular prescription', was sold as explicitly following the University [of Pennsylvania] Pharmacy formulation (arsenous acid, strychnine sulphate, cinchonine sulphate, iron carbonate and extract of belladonna)[127] and Mulford's Rhubarb and Ipecac preparation originated at the Roosevelt Hospital.[128] When research was undertaken at Mulford on bacterins, a large number of cultures were gathered from Philadelphia hospitals by Mulford staff.[129] Eighty strains were grown for testing after 115 had been collected during the winter of 1910.

Private physicians were usually cooperative as well, even when not paid by the company to publicise their product. Edwin Rosenthal tested Mulford's diphtheria antitoxin a number of times during the first year of its production, tallying its record against its competitors. He found that in its first full year of use Mulford's was as popular as Behring's preparation imported from Hoechst. The actual results of clinical trials were not conclusive but did indicate that the domestic product was comparable to the original German antitoxin.[130]

Most of the flow of information, innovation and technique passed from academic institutions into the company laboratory. Some of it was channelled through informal contacts, some through licensing and some through a concerted effort by employees to bring valuable information to Mulford. Dr W. F. Elgin, who joined Mulford from the National Vaccine Establishment to work on smallpox vaccine in 1898, travelled widely to gather ideas for consideration at Glenolden. Under the joint auspices of the company and the Board of Health of Pennsylvania, he visited vaccine laboratories in England, Belgium, France, Germany, Switzerland and Italy. While investigating methods for the collection of pus for smallpox vaccine, he noted, for example, that:

> the one thing of prime importance was observed in Cologne where calves are killed just prior to removal of the pulp. This method was adopted upon my return and resulted in nearly doubling the output per calf.[131]

Close collaboration with universities was one of Milton Campbell's main interests. He attributed much of the greatness of pre-war German science to this cooperation, aided by limitations in German patent law which allowed coverage only of processes and apparatus relating to foods, chemicals and medicines, leaving products open to competition.[132] The company encouraged this type of cooperation by fostering goodwill as best it could. It offered a prize at the Philadelphia College of Pharmacy for outstanding students in pharmacology[133] and hosted the American Chemical Society on a visit in 1919.[134] Whenever friendly cooperation failed to bring university-developed products to Mulford, they were willing to purchase production rights. Tethelin, a product of the pituitary gland used to promote wound healing, was developed at the University of California. Mulford arranged to produce Tethelin under licence, agreeing to pay royalties to the university, which acted as assignee.[135]

Various means were used to strengthen ties between the company and the medical community. Salesmen were trained to present 'details' of new products to members of the community, from the highest to the lowest. In one report by the company, the success of such a 'detail man' was vividly illustrated.

> We take this opportunity of passing along some information and suggestions recently obtained by one of our representatives, Mr. J. C. Peacock, in his detail work with the dentists and dental colleges in Philadelphia. Contact with the leading members of the faculties of the Philadelphia Dental College and of the University of Pennsylvania Dental School, revealed that they were already 'sold'. In both institutions, Hypo-Units were in use and members of the faculties were interested in having their students, and dentists generally, become better acquainted with this unique injecting device. . . . One of the faculty members pointed out that the teaching they received during their college course will determine, largely, what the students will use when they start in practice for themselves. For this reason, they welcomed the opportunity to acquaint their students with Hypo-Units, and suggested that pocket cases be provided for demonstration and for display at the school.[136]

Providing such devices as the 'Hypo-Units' was performing a kind of service for the medical profession. By the war, Mulford was offering services which, on the surface, seemed even less connected with commercial endeavour. In April 1918 a new service was discussed at Mulford's executive meeting concerning the:

> desirability of our quietly interesting our leading distributors in making arrangements to do laboratory work for physicians, such as making diagnostic tests, differentiating types of infection, etc. . . .[137]

This service had two business purposes, the first was to make better use of the staff and extensive laboratories possessed by the company. In addition, 'any druggist who shows the proper activity and knowledge in this direction will naturally secure the bulk of the biological business in his entire community'.[138] Diagnostic services opened a large area for the firm with little extra effort. Samples were collected in pharmacies and sent through the mail or by company representatives back to Glenolden. There the experimental laboratories could easily be used for routine testing and within a few years an inexpensive service was available for the diagnosis of a dozen infectious diseases, along with general services such as urinalysis. A 'complete hay fever service' was offered to complement Mulford's extensive offerings of pollen extracts.[139] It was then hoped that therapies could be supplied to the physicians who sent specimens to be tested. However, such services benefited the medical community as well as the company, and strengthened the ties between them.

Mulford was held in good repute by pharmacologists, at a time when the legitimacy of academic pharmacologists' affiliations with drug houses was being questioned. The Society for Pharmacology and Experimental Therapeutics had explicitly forbidden any members to work for drug companies,[140] a prohibition taken very seriously by academic pharmacologists. They recognised that in order to establish a legitimate professional identity on the same level with, for example, physiologists, they needed to cleanse themselves of their image as pharmacists, patent medicine makers or hired hands used for scientific endorsements. Mulford secured their support by agreeing with their position. Pharmacy, Dr Gould argued in the *Mulford Digest*, should become a medical specialty:

> Cooperation on the part of the medical and pharmaceutical professions and of manufacturers engaged in the pharmacal and chemical industries will largely help in bringing this about.[141]

After all, he continued:

> As practitioners of the pharmacologic arts we are provided with laboratories for research and manufacturing purposes. We employ chemists, botanists, pharmacists, pharmacologists, to direct the laboratories and the publication of our literature.[142]

Scientists had every reason for wishing to maintain their contacts with firms such as Mulford. It was through them that they were given elaborate facilities and opportunities for research, which their somewhat marginal position in the medical world often denied them elsewhere. A typical experience in a commercial laboratory was related by Selman Waksman, later well-known for his research on antibiotics. While a graduate student in microbiology at the University of California before the war, he was offered part-time work while studying.

I was in charge of the biochemistry department. My job consisted in supervising a group of some ten or fifteen men and women who were preparing various media for the growth of different organisms.[143]

While at the Cutter Laboratory he worked on antitoxins, vaccines and serums, was able to use their laboratory facilities for some of his own research and in 1917 developed a new type of peptone for the production of diphtheria antitoxin.[144]

The company was not oblivious to its good fortune in being situated in a great medical centre:

with our extensive professional and commercial affiliations at home and abroad, we are advantageously placed for obtaining information. . . .[145]

The close and amicable relations which Mulford fostered with universities, hospitals, pharmacologists and leading physicians in private practice served the company well in its rapid expansion in the years before the war.

MULFORD PEAKS

In the first decade of the twentieth century, diphtheria antitoxin continued to be Mulford's most profitable product.[146] Two major problems in its production, short shelf-life and low potency, had largely been resolved. There had been no method for concentrating diphtheria antitoxin until 1900, and the large doses administered often created pain and distress. Continuing efforts were made to manufacture stronger solutions and after the first year of its production, the potency began to double annually.[147] In 1900 and working in collaboration with the company, Torald Sollmann solved these problems with a technique which isolated the antitoxic bodies from their associated serum globulins. Sollmann, a prominent pharmacologist at Western Reserve University in Cleveland, perfected a method of crystallising the blood serum and developed a technique for concentrating antitoxin. This procedure also lengthened the shelf-life up to six weeks:

A more extended and careful study of the animals producing antitoxic serum, and an increased strength in the diphtheria toxin given them, have enabled us to produce Antitoxin of many times our former standard strength; while, at the same time, improvements in the methods of preserving the serum have enabled us to prevent almost entirely the urticaria [hives] and other untoward effects formerly ascribed to antitoxic serums.[148]

This change consequently allowed the company to advertise antitoxin as an item which could be stocked in pharmacies, rather than ordered for immediate use.[149]

Mulford acquired an early lead in supplying diphtheria antitoxin to city boards of health which either did not produce their own antitoxin or fell short of their needs.[150] Lederle Laboratories, however, were able to secure a number of contracts on account of their close ties to the New York City Board of Health. Lederle also sold to the Philadelphia Board during the long period when the city refused it sufficient appropriations to build an efficient laboratory.[151] The company also began to secure contracts from other large city departments. In 1907, for example, Lederle made substantial sales to the state boards of health in Ohio, Minnesota, Kentucky, Maryland and Illinois as well as smaller sales to Rhode Island. Though the contract negotiations cannot be charted, one suspects that the animosity the Philadelphia Board felt towards Joseph McFarland after his departure to Mulford was the main reason that the company lost the bid for such a relatively large, steady and local customer. H. M. Alexander had perhaps the largest number of contracts with state boards of health by the end of the war, selling some of its diphtheria and tetanus antitoxins to most states in the Union.[152] Mulford was losing its early advantage to its new competitors.

Partly because of the threat to its diphtheria antitoxin market, and partly because of the promise that other biological drugs would produce similarly remarkable profits, Mulford turned increasingly to their development. In 1905 Simon Flexner began a series of experiments at the Rockefeller Institute with a serum he devised with toxin from meningococcic cultures.[153] Following the procedure for diphtheria antitoxin of injecting horses and separating and concentrating the serum, he tested the product in 1905–06 among the full range of experimental animals and in 1908–09 extended this to humans.[154] Flexner's clinical results were inconclusive but encouraging, although there were continuing problems with the classical bacteriological analysis of meningitis. Mulford was sufficiently convinced, however, that the antimeningitis serum had great potential.

> Mr. Campbell approved a suggestion . . . that we particularly push the sale of such serums as are not made and distributed generally by State Boards of Health, etc., always emphasizing the superiority of Mulford products. Antimeningococcic Serum was cited as an example. . . . Mr. Campbell asked Dr. Reichal to make it a point to send us important laboratory facts, which we might later dress up and utilize for sales work.[155]

The antimeningitis serum sold well in the succeeding years, although it hardly affected the morbidity and mortality rates. Mulford began marketing the serum as early as 1910, amidst conflicting epidemiological data. Even after the decision was made, it was promoted with advertisements which were slightly more restrained than those for other biologicals. The company stressed that the treatment should begin as soon after the onset of symptoms as possible, that sufficient doses must be used, and warned that 'although the serum is ordinarily without benefit in chronic cases, it may occasionally do good'.[156] In the winter of 1912–13, during an outbreak of cerebrospinal meningitis in Dyer County, Tennessee, Mulford's serum was extensively used. As with other epidemiological reports of meningitis, the findings were mixed, but the medicine performed sufficiently well to warrant the episode being presented in advertisements.[157]

A second edition of *Working Bulletin Number 8* was offered in 1917, advertising improvements in the serum and giving information on the treatment of meningitis.

> After a thorough study of all the well-known procedures with their complicated details, means have been evolved in the Mulford Laboratories by which the most advanced methods of treating cerebrospinal fever may be simplified and thus placed at the disposal of the physician.[158]

In this revision, the 'relative failure'[159] of the treatment was 'readily explained'.[160] Four distinct serological types of meningococcus were identified and systematic tests by Gordon in England described to confirm that serum produced by one of these types was not potent against the others. With this information at hand, the company could assure physicians that with the proper serological identification, their treatment would be effective. Mulford even offered an explanation for the few instances when serum treatment seemed effective by suggesting that in some cases there was, by coincidence, a high ratio of correspondence between serum and serological type.[161]

New techniques of diagnosis were recommended with specimens taken from the mouth and nose, in addition to the spine. Mulford provided full details on culturing the cocci and testing the agglutination (for serological type). Ordering instructions were also provided, with careful specification of the appropriate serum type. As with other *Working Bulletins* after 1912, a notice was conspicuously attached which warned that:

> different brands of pharmaceutical and biological products differ widely in regard to their therapeutic value. This variation accounts for many of the failures to secure results from the administration of established remedies.[162]

When, in 1938, long-term epidemiological studies of cerebrospinal meningitis were published, it became clear that there had been no difference, over all, in the pre-serum and post-serum years. As one researcher then wrote:

> It is my opinion from the available evidence that the treatment of epidemic cerebrospinal meningitis as used in the urban population described over the time period to which I have had reference has reduced the fatality of this disease little if at all.[163]

Mulford's visible application of scientific theories and practice, however, promoted its success. Output at Mulford began to rise with the rapid growth of military forces in Europe in 1914.[164] Milton Campbell secured the largest single contract for the company when he was able to convince the medical supply officers of the army that they could simplify their purchasing arrangements for diphtheria antitoxin and be assured of good quality if they gave Mulford an exclusive contract. Campbell took a considerable risk in seeking this contract, since he was staking the company's production capacity on meeting this one huge order. He immediately began a programme of expansion which brought the size of the diphtheria antitoxin sector to 1500 horses and 1200 employees.[165] In little over twenty years, the H. K. Mulford Company had built itself upon a scientific basis – in technique as in management – from a small pharmacy to a major industrial force.

6 Science-based Industry: Scientific Disputes and Government Regulation

By the first decade of the twentieth century, many American pharmaceutical firms had become science-based, not merely associated in a superficial way with science. Many of their products emerged from the laboratory and they conducted their advertising campaigns in scientific terms. Their disputes were necessarily waged on a new level, carried on in terms that laymen could not ordinarily follow. They would, for example, call into question the laboratory facilities or the method of production of a competitor's wares. Science was now used to define whether a company had attained an appropriately high level of quality.

This period also saw new involvement by government in the pharmaceutical industry, in the form of the 1902 and 1906 Acts regulating drug production. Companies had fought state intervention in the shape of the public health boards' production of antitoxins, but many approved this new involvement. In particular, the larger, more scientifically advanced welcomed it because it gave legal definition to the substance of their disputes: it defined the level of scientific equipment and expertise that any firm must have. It therefore served to 'rationalise' the industry, forcing out of business the small producers who could not afford to equip themselves satisfactorily. The number of companies competing in the marketplace therefore declined.

DISPUTE AMONG EXPERTS: CONTAMINATED VACCINE IN CAMDEN

In 1901 an outbreak of tetanus occurred in Camden, New Jersey, an incident seemingly connected to contaminated smallpox vaccine. The subsequent dispute over the incident polarised opinion about the one major change made in vaccine production since Edward Jenner – the introduction of glycerinated lymph. Two commercial vaccine producers figured largely in the argument, the H. K. Mulford Company and H. M. Alexander's Vaccine Farm. Accusations were hurled by all concerned, hardly a new phenomenon. Their novelty, however, lay in the scientific form they now took.

Since Jenner's time smallpox vaccine had either been passed arm to arm, or prepared by taking material from the cowpox vesicles of cattle and transferring them to some inoculating instrument.[1] By the 1880s the preparation of dry points had been developed as a commercially feasible technique.[2] The vaccine material was taken in small quantities from a heifer, transferred to ivory points and allowed to dry before being packaged.[3] Glycerinated lymph was developed in 1897 to preserve and dilute the vaccine before it was transferred to sealed glass tubes.[4]

About eighty cases of tetanus occurred in Camden in late 1901.[5] An immediate public association was made between the cases and smallpox vaccination, soon focusing on glycerinated lymph as a probable cause of the outbreak. Joseph McFarland, who had left the H. K. Mulford Company for a professorship at the Medico-Chirurgical College and a position with Parke Davis, investigated their causes, and explored any links with smallpox vaccinations.[6] He collected information on eleven of the cases that occurred in November and found that in every instance the outbreak of the disease post-dated inoculation by three to four weeks and that in ten of the cases glycerinated virus had been used. Dry virus had been used in the eleventh case.[7]

McFarland's former employer, Mulford, was clearly implicated by the findings.[8] Mulford's glycerinated vaccines seemed to be most closely connected with the tetanus cases. The firm sold both dry and glycerinated preparations, but recommended the latter, citing the preference of thirty-one 'well-known authorities' including George M. Sternberg (Surgeon General, US Army), Walter C. Wyman (Surgeon General, US Marine Hospital Service), Walter Reed, Theobald Smith, William H. Park and William M. Welch.[9] Mulford's vaccine was implicated in forty of the seventy-seven cases of tetanus in 1901.[10]

Mulford's name was immediately associated with these cases because it claimed to have substantial sales of smallpox vaccine in the Camden area. Other firms were soon implicated, too, because of their previous claims.[11] Mulford and its competitors all advertised that their products were widely used, giving sales figures which are hard to verify or contradict. Both Mulford and H. M. Alexander marketed a great deal in eastern Pennsylvania and New Jersey, although, of the two firms, Mulford probably secured more contracts with public health departments and greater sales to druggists.[12] Mulford's greater success now made it the focus for the controversy over contaminated vaccine. The stand Mulford chose was to stress Alexander's role, a charge which the latter hotly denied.

A grudge between the two companies had existed from the early 1890s when Henry Mulford had asked to join Dr Alexander in a partnership.[13] Alexander refused his offer, arguing that he himself had a monopoly on the vaccine business which he was not prepared to relinquish. Mulford's rivalry with Alexander was heightened by this rejection.

In the 1901 cases, Mulford held that two New Jersey pharmacists, agents and representatives of Parke Davis and of H. M. Alexander, were responsible for suggesting that Mulford's product had been used and that it must have been contaminated. George M. Beringer, a Camden druggist, had written to the local newspaper naming Mulford and directly accusing the firm of causing nine of the deaths. W. Pitt Rich, a Parke Davis employee, distributed copies of this letter. Beringer, a 'special agent' of Parke Davis, was, according to Mulford:

> formerly a debtor to our company for a considerable sum, and was compelled to pay the account by due process of law shortly before the publication of his letter.[14]

He had further cause besides this alleged grudge for wishing to malign Mulford: he had apparently been trying to secure contracts from both Parke Davis and H. M. Alexander to supply their vaccine to Camden's Public Health Department, 'which business, however, was secured by ourselves [Mulford] on account of the superiority of our product'.

The arguments soon shifted, however, from accusations of personal animosity to the scientific reliability of the vaccine itself. Mulford's opponents focused on its use of glycerinated lymph, which the company had claimed as a mark of scientific advancement. Mulford claimed its competitors were attempting to discredit this method of vaccine preparation for commercial not scientific reasons, using the outbreak of tetanus as their excuse. Behind it all, Mulford suggested, H. M. Alexander, working in collaboration with Parke Davis, had established a front, the Pennsylvania Vaccine Company.[15]

Most of the smaller vaccine farms were owned and operated by physicians. This was true of Dr Slee's Pocono Laboratories, Dr

Walsh's National Vaccine Establishment, Dr Alexander's Lancaster County Vaccine Farms, the Cutter Laboratories in San Francisco, and numerous others in the mid-west.[16] As small businesses, they routinely concerned themselves with cultivating their local markets and were, therefore, typical of the companies which the larger firms like Mulford sought to eliminate. The Pennsylvania Vaccine Farm was not subsequently licensed by the government, which perhaps supports Mulford's charges as to its low standards.[17] Mulford pointed out that the Pennsylvania State Board of Health had thoroughly condemned this farm in 1896: 'this establishment', the Board had argued:

> has rather a commercial than a scientific aspect. It is very doubtful if ashes have any disinfecting properties, such as is claimed by the operator. The fact that the hay-loft is directly over the incubating stables renders it possible to have very dirty and infected vesicles, since dust can filter down upon the backs of the animals. No tuberculin is used. Cattle seem thin and scrubby. The separate charging of the points by hand and laying them in a dirty plate is neither clean nor hygienic. It is doubtful if a wooden paddle can be thoroughly cleaned, and its use in removing pus should be discontinued, since it is likely to infect fairly healthy vesicles, if such exist. The mattress-covered operating racks are filthy.[19]

The vaccine farm dated back to 1874, but was only incorporated after 1901. Mulford claimed that it had been bought by H. M. Alexander. Its stock, Mulford argued, was owned by George R. Heisey, an attorney for Alexander. Mulford also accused the farm of deliberately misleading its customers: it had falsely claimed to have distributed a letter which said: 'We have been seriously considering the question of ceasing the propagation of glycerinized vaccine: we entered into it much against our better judgment.'[20] Mulford argued that the Pennsylvania Vaccine Farm had never used glycerinated vaccine, but always dry points. It seemed that if it were now a front for Alexander, it was being used to discredit Mulford's method of making vaccine while Alexander could continue to associate itself with the scientifically advanced glycerinated lymph.[21] The distinction between the two forms of vaccine is significant. Arguments were based both on commercial and scientific grounds and the comparative strength of the latter is shown by the emphasis given it in the rhetoric of the controversy. The contrast in the language Mulford used to describe the bacteriologically sophisticated means used to produce glycerinated vaccine with the 'crude' and 'unsterile' methods employed by producers of dry points, was intended to accentuate their difference.

> The purpose of glycerinized lymph is to starve out such pathogenic organisms as are invariably found in vaccine when it is first collected and, also, to make all the vaccine glycerinized and triturated of uniform consistency and activity. Glycerin does not impair the value of the vaccine, but does starve out other organisms.[22]

Mulford described the production of dry points as a much cruder procedure, stressing that the immediate transfer of virus from heifer to vaccine point was unsanitary.

> . . . all the germs and inflammatory products which are necessarily present in and about the vaccinated area of the heifer are, from very necessity, transferred direct to the ivory point. Consequently, vaccine points can never be absolutely free from germs and dangerous foreign material (necrosed tissue). Furthermore, the points cannot be tested for activity.[23]

H. M. Alexander publicly came to the defence of glycerinated vaccine, stressing its proven reliability. The technique was, he argued, much older than McFarland, for instance, seemed to think.[24] As he wrote to McFarland,

> I have just read your address as printed in the American Medical Journal [sic] and note what you say with regard to Dr. Copeman of London having discovered and advocated the use of Glycerinized Lymph in 1891, referring to it as so many others have done as a new thing. Now I made it in this manner myself in 1882 and every year since, out of the third source of course, not using the impurities; and I purchased it from different Establishments in this country back as early as 1876. Every Vaccine producer in Europe had made it long before I began the business in 1882, and have continued to thus produce it mixed with Glycerine and distilled water ever since. I cannot find just now the histories to enable me to say with a certainty just how many years ago it was thus produced; but my recollection is that it goes back over half a century.[25]

Of course, the difference in the claims made for vaccine produced with glycerine before and after the 1890s was the use of bacteriological theory to explain its properties. This was expressed by Alexander in a later letter when he specified that:

I and others added Glycerine in the proportion of from 33 1/3 to 66 2/3%. . . . It may have been that it was added by some for the absolute purpose of preserving it. I beg to say that I discussed the matter of the discovery of certain bacteria with Dr. Stephen C. Martin before Copeman's supposed discovery [1891] and I also discussed it with one other propagator before that time, as well as a number of eminent medical authorities.

The question which I asked as far back as 1887 was this. While Glycerine seems to purify Vaccine Lymph, as well as preserve it, why is its action still not as true and perfect as its protection equal to that of Dried Virus. The only thing that I can see is that since Copeman told the world that it would do this, that parties have engaged in the sale of all the dirty stuff they could gather up, depending on the Glycerine to save them.[26]

Whatever role Alexander was playing behind the scenes in urging small vaccine producers who used dry points to attack Mulford, his public face seemed above reproach.

Mulford now contended that the negative publicity glycerinated vaccine was still receiving would endanger the public image of vaccination as a whole, and provide fuel for antivaccinationists. In this way it hoped to associate itself with enlightened opinion, and to suggest that its competitors were merely conservative pill pushers. Mulford also allied itself with well-established, enlightened opinion by distributing the 'Official Report of the Camden Board of Health Concerning the Cases of Tetanus Which Occurred in Patients who had been Vaccinated'.[27] The report cited 'indisputable evidence' that vaccination was not to blame, and gave the board's own account of how vaccination had led indirectly to tetanus.[28] First of all, the vaccines were clearly not contaminated. The outbreak of tetanus would have occurred five to nine days after exposure, and the cases in question all developed three to five weeks after vaccination. Furthermore, samples from all the batches of Mulford's vaccine had been obtained, usually from local druggists, and none proved contaminated. What was likely, it argued, was that the open sores from the vaccinations had become infected. 'Tetanus, or any other infection, can never occur if the vaccination is properly protected from contact with the atmosphere or with soiled clothing, bandages, etc.'[29]

In order to explain the incidence of tetanus in Camden, the report turned to a well-accepted combination of bacteriology and meteorology, logically presented in an amalgam of plausible reasons:

The tetanus cases in Camden are to be explained upon atmospheric and telluric conditions which have prevailed in Camden during the past six weeks. There had been a long period of dry weather with high winds, so that tetanus germs, which have their normal habitat in the earth dust, dirt of stables, etc., have been constantly distributed in the atmosphere. It is noticeable in all the cases, after careful examination as to cause, that the wound had been exposed by the scab being knocked off or removed, or else the arm had been injured and infection resulted; frequently children scratched the vaccinated area with their dirty fingers and nails and infected the wound.[30]

With the corroboration of bacteriological examinations of suspected virus by the New Jersey State Board of Health and the Cooper Hospital, Camden, the Camden City Board of Health rested its case.[31] It also had further support from the Philadelphia Board of Health, which had vaccinated 100 000 people with commercial preparations in the preceding three months, as well as reassurance from elsewhere, including the Surgeon General's Office.[32]

This report did not silence public outcry. The coincidence of vaccination followed by tetanus seemed too significant. As Dr Ralph Walsh, proprietor of the National Vaccine Establishment in Washington, DC, wrote:

I am inclined to believe that the New Jersey cases were due to after infection and that the vaccine was not at fault, yet the fact that the cases in Philadelphia, Camden and Atlantic City occurred almost simultaneously and from vaccine propagated by the same party staggers me.[33]

McFarland undertook further research on the matter, collecting 119 cases of tetanus after inoculation stretching from 1839 to 1902, seventy-seven of which occurred in 1901, mostly in southern New Jersey and eastern Pennsylvania.[34] Using H. M. Alexander as one of his sources, he found that six cases of tetanus following vaccination occurred 'around Washington in 1892' and therefore might have originated in Walsh's laboratory. Although Walsh was adamant that this was not the case, Alexander maintained his point.[35] Alexander also cited cases of tetanus which led to deaths in Cleveland, Los Angeles, Fall River and elsewhere, claiming to McFarland that the Cleveland cases at least 'followed the use of Mulford's and Stearn's [vaccines]'.[36]

Besides implicating Mulford's products, Alexander's citation of

Walsh's vaccine, brought in another major merchant.[37] Walsh had used glycerinated lymph for a number of years, largely to counteract the constant problem of inactive vaccine. This was the major reason for using glycerine until 1891, when Monkton Copeman's article appeared in London and gave additional, bacteriological reasons for using glycerinated lymph.[38] Walsh now entered the controversy, not only defending glycerinated lymph, but also claiming precedence in its use. He stated that the Laboratories of the National Vaccine Establishment were 'the first to recommend the use of glycerinized lymph to the Profession of the United States'.[39]

The dispute over glycerinated versus dry lymph quickly evolved into a reassessment of corporate responsibility. If the vaccines had been contaminated then the blame rested on the unsanitary practices of the producer. However, if one form of inoculating instrument or preparation was inherently less safe than the other, then the responsibility would have to be shared with the purchaser and perhaps the market as a whole. Despite the official Camden report that had identified infected scabs as the cause, sharing the blame between the inoculating physicians and the patient would mean exonerating the producers completely. The public health boards needed to protect their vaccination policy. At the same time they could ill afford to deny the correlation between inoculated children and tetanus. They resorted to a defence of their policy and their suppliers, but in addition emphasised their role as guides and supervisors of local doctors. In the meantime the companies involved, particularly Mulford and Alexander, continued to battle over each other's accusations.

Alexander's response to Mulford's pamphlet was presented to McFarland in his continuing role as investigator of the incidents. It contained a complete refutation of Mulford's accusations.[40] Graciously pointing out that he had not taken advantage of Mulford's 'uncomfortable situation', Alexander felt particularly disappointed that they should come out with 'a pamphlet which is false in every particular'.[41] Against the specific accusation by Mulford that he owned stock in the Pennsylvania Vaccine Farm, Alexander countered that 'Mulford was dickering for some stock'[42] in the farm. Other statements in the pamphlet were contradicted, and the consequence of the affair, Alexander argued, boded well for his company. He claimed that where they had shown 'what consumate liars these people have proven themselves', by Alexander's pamphlet, physicians had shown great animosity both towards 'their operations [and] their statements', and 'we have had Boards of Health come solidly to us and drop the use of

Mulford's goods'. Alexander went on to note 'the benefits accruing to us' as a result of this contretemps.[43]

McFarland's preliminary report on the Camden outbreak had been presented to the Philadelphia County Medical Society in late November.[44] In it he had implied that only Mulford vaccine was involved. Mulford responded with the criticism that McFarland had defended his current employer, Parke Davis, while implicating his previous one. It also suggested that McFarland should 'have this rectified at the earliest moment so as to prevent this error appearing in the Medical Journals'.[45] Dr Charles Hofer of Mulford conducted an investigation into the outbreak of tetanus, under the direction of Milton Campbell, and claimed to have identified all the vaccines used in Camden during the outbreak. Some cases, he argued, occurred after the use of Alexander's vaccine, but he insisted that in any event none had been caused by vaccination. They were all secondary infections. Thus H. K. Mulford could himself write to McFarland:

> The writer would consider it a very unwise undertaking for you to endeavor to prove that the vaccine caused tetanus until you have examined the virus yourself, and thinks that you have been unwise in making any statement that might be taken up by the lay journals, giving the impression that vaccine caused tetanus, especially in view of the fact that the entire country is threatened with an epidemic of smallpox. . . .[46]

The implication in Mulford's letter was that, for the public good, it would be best to remain silent on the scientific assessments of various methods of vaccination, lest laymen reacted against inoculation altogether. He implied, therefore, that there was a realm of scientific inquiry that the layman should not enter.

AFTERMATH OF THE CAMDEN INCIDENT

The episode in Camden had revealed disputes within the industry, which, although hardly unprecedented were couched in the new terms of science. Partly as a result of such incidents, the issue of government control arose; biological standards could not be determined by market forces alone. Efforts to improve the quality of smallpox vaccine were not working. The 1901 cases of tetanus came in the midst of a smallpox epidemic that spanned 1900–02.[47]

As a response to the poor showing of the producers, and no doubt aggravated by their rivalry, the Massachusetts State Board argued that protection could only be guaranteed if the state supervised the preparation of vaccine lymph.[48] Theobald Smith, who had worked his way to a position of commanding authority as director of the Massachusetts State laboratories, argued that since vaccine was very perishable, the state must oversee its supply in order to protect the programme of compulsory vaccination. In 1903 he even went as far as to petition the state government for funds for the laboratories' own production of smallpox vaccine as was already the case with diphtheria antitoxin.[49]

With threats that the state governments might fund the production of vaccine as they had antitoxin, the manufacturers had at least to feign decisive action. Advertising and close contacts with physicians and public health bodies became crucial. Some firms realised this even while their efforts to supply vaccine during the epidemic were clearly failing. The most common form of advertising consisted of the collection and reprinting of testimonials by physician users. This approach was used extensively by Pocono Laboratories, producers of Slee's glycerinated vaccine virus.[50] Dr Richard Slee ran a small operation, but boasted of major sales to the United States Army, some provincial governments in Canada and some US state boards of health, including those of Pennsylvania, Illinois and Nebraska.[51] Not surprisingly, he considered it crucial that the acrimonious debates over glycerinated vaccine should not prejudice his customers against it.

The public wariness which resulted from the outbreaks of tetanus and the squabble between the companies contributed to an upsurge in antivaccinationist activity. Antivaccinationist sentiment had grown during each of the previous smallpox outbreaks and, though its impact was limited, it did concern the companies sufficiently to provoke responses. 'Vaccination is safe' became the message now hurriedly presented by the companies as well as by public health advocates. It was received by the public with the usual reservations, but the companies involved were later more hesitant to bring their disputes into the public arena.[52]

In their efforts to re-establish equilibrium and continue their battles over appropriate standards for new medicines, the three leading producers, Mulford, Alexander and Parke Davis shifted their dispute to safer terrain. With minor producers creating competitive difficulties, the leading vaccine manufacturers directed their attacks against unsanitary and outmoded laboratories. For this a new forum had to be found and it was to Washington that they now turned.

REGULATION: THE 1902 ACT

With the stimulus of public concern after the affair in Camden and a parallel incident in St Louis, Congress bowed to lobbyists in 1902 and passed an act to control the production and sale of biologicals, and to regulate the sale of viruses, serums, toxins and analogous products.[53] The act specified that manufacturers must be licensed by the Secretary of the Treasury (through the Laboratory of Hygiene) and each package of vaccine must be properly labelled and dated. It also allowed for 'reasonable inspection' of company properties at any time and provided guidelines for enforcement of action against unsatisfactory firms.[54]

Inspection and licensing began immediately, with the major producers competing to obtain licences as soon as possible. By the end of 1902 the first had been obtained by Parke Davis, the second by H. K. Mulford, and the third by H. M. Alexander's Vaccine Farm.[55] Licences were soon granted to seven other pharmaceutical and chemical firms, including the Pasteur Institute (Paris) and the Berlin manufacturer Chemische Fabrik auf Aktien (E. Schering).[56]

For the first time the manufacturers of biologicals had to face drug regulation in its modern form. Their relationships with each other and with the government changed, and they developed a new attitude towards their products. Regulation of vaccine and antitoxin producers created a much more coherent competitive group. Each company could easily find out through the Hygienic Laboratory which other firms around the country were producing similar products and it was then easy to establish the relative quality of their competitors' wares. A more settled pattern of competition was brought to the major producers through the standards set by the Hygienic Laboratory. Regulation also strengthened the ties between government laboratories and academic pharmacologists, bacteriologists and pathologists. The government became one of the most significant conduits through which academic scientists could enter the profitable corporate world; the 'revolving door' which circulated people between the government regulatory agencies and the companies they regulated established itself soon after the laws were put into effect.[57]

The Hygienic Laboratory grew out of the predecessor to the Public Health service, the Marine Hospital Service.[58] Bacteriological investigations in the Service began at the Marine Hospital building at Stapleton, Staten Island, New York, where Joseph Kinyoun established a 'laboratory of hygiene' in August 1887.[59] When he moved with the laboratory to Washington, his bacteriological work was expanded somewhat through the production of diphtheria antitoxin in 1895. By 1902 the laboratory had developed considerable expertise in the assessment of biologicals.

The 1902 Act stimulated the growth of the Hygienic Laboratory. The regular staff included inspectors who visited the vaccine and antitoxin farms, laboratory personnel who monitored samples, and a large clerical staff which processed licence applications, renewals and the appeals of rejected manufacturers.[60] The staff came to know the leading companies well. Standards were often set by assessing the abilities of the leading producers to maintain a certain level of purity or concentration or follow a particularly safe laboratory procedure. Kinyoun, for example, visited the Mulford Company frequently and used its methods both to check other producers' antitoxins and vaccines and to help set guidelines for concentration and toxicity for the industry as a whole.[61] His contacts with the company continued after he was succeeded by Milton Rosenau as director of the Laboratory in 1899. Kinyoun continued to work for the Public Health Service until 1903 when he resigned to join Mulford as head of the Glenolden plant and director of biologicals production.[62]

An incident in 1908 illuminates how the Laboratory exercised the powers of the 1902 Act. In that year an outbreak of hoof and mouth disease was discovered in the Parke Davis vaccine herd and in their antitoxin stables.[63] The product from the infected and exposed animals was immediately taken off the market and the company's licence was temporarily suspended. The disease continued to spread and reached the Mulford farm within weeks. The carrier was not discovered, but it is possible that either an inspector transmitted the disease, or even that the companies, rivals though they were, could have exchanged animals. Mulford's licence was also suspended. Both companies quickly complied with the recommendations of the Laboratory and eradicated the disease. In the meantime they were constantly monitored both to assure satisfactory progress in complying with their clean-up efforts and to guard against any contaminated products reaching the market. They were allowed to resume production after about five months.[64]

REGULATION: THE 1906 ACT

The 1906 Pure Food and Drugs Act was a response to the growing demand that state regulations be standardised, along with various special interest pressures ranging from large drug manufacturers such as Smith Kline and French to the pleading of Harvey Wiley at the Department of Agriculture.[65] Similar bills had been submitted to Congress since the 1890s and a number of hearings had been held on the proposals for uniform regulations controlling drug labelling and marketing.[66] The main thrust of the bill was to control the adulteration of food, Harvey Wiley's main goal, rather than regulate drugs.

The act swept through Congress after the public outcry following Upton Sinclair's novel, *The Jungle*, and it was the food adulterators that Wiley zealously pursued.[67] Not that offenders such as Durham's Pure Leaf Lard Company, Sinclair's fictitious version of meat packers, were prosecuted, but rather the smaller producers whom Wiley considered irresponsible. Similarly with drug makers, the large manufacturers, were not indicted. Many had, indeed, supported the bill.[68]

Mahlon N. Kline, vice-president of Smith Kline and French and an active lobbyist in Washington, presented in 1905, 'Some Reasons Why The Internal Revenue Tax on Alcohol Should be Reduced, and Why our Government Should Provide Free Denaturized Alcohol for use in the Arts'.[69] Mahlon Kline's Washington work brought him into contact with Harvey Wiley, chief of the Bureau of Chemistry. Wiley had for many years been agitating for legislation for the regulation of foods and adulteration of drugs. He may have been surprised by the enthusiastic support he received from Mahlon Kline for proposals to regulate the quality of drugs, but the company's position was clear: they wished to exploit to the full their near monopoly on certain markets and the facilities of their laboratory.[70] Mahlon Kline's activities in Washington may have been no more than a convenience for Harvey Wiley, but to the leaders of the drug trade his work renewed the possibility of reducing competition by driving smaller producers out. As head of the National Wholesale Druggists Association and chairman of its committee on legislation, he was considered 'the most influential man in the drug industry'.[71] It was important, then, that he believed that the new law would become:

the greatest instrument for the moral uplifting of the average businessman that had ever been bestowed upon the American people.[72]

The 1906 Act was primarily intended to provide the Department of Agriculture with the legal power to enforce reasonable standards of purity for processed foods. It included provisions for inspection of processing facilities and analysis of foods. It also specified that certain main ingredients had to be identified on package labels and that the labels could not be misleading.[73] It extended the law covering imports of tea (1883), and of foods, drugs and liquors (1890).[74] The administration of the drug regulations in the 1906 Act fell on Lyman Kebler, who was no longer with Smith Kline and French, but had become chief of the Drug Laboratory in the Department of Agriculture's Bureau of Chemistry.[75] Court action under the law could bring cessation order, confiscation and destruction of stocks, and a fine. Very few of the early cases were brought against drug makers or pharmacists, despite numerous flagrant abuses, and those which were resulted in small fines.[76]

Kebler's office was in charge of a growing staff of chemists and clerical assistants whose first task was to determine the boundary between drugs and food, for which different criteria were enforced. During the first year of the act, 600 items were examined, 107 of which were chemical reagents, 70 were samples of hops tested for arsenic, and the rest various raw drugs and patent medicines. The drugs tested included a large amount of cod-liver oil.[77]

The main purpose of the regulatory work was meant, however, to be the control of patent medicines, many of which were obtained from the Post Office Department for inspection as items sent through the mail.[78] In the second year of its enforcement the drug inspection was expanded from Kebler's laboratory to an entire Division of Drugs which had the capacity to inspect a much larger sample than previously. In addition to the now routine inspection of patent medicines, the division tested a large number of chemical reagents, soft drinks and medicinal oils. Crude drugs were also inspected in the laboratory, with special attention given to imported medicines.[79]

Extensive cooperation with the American Medical Asspciation and the Post Office was maintained during the first years of the act. The AMA in particular wished to expose patent medicine frauds and published the results of the joint investigations in its *Journal*.[80] The Post Office used the Bureau in its efforts to control fraud through the mail.

Within a few years the effects of the inspections were evident. Shipments of belladonna root, for example, had commonly been found to be contaminated by foreign roots, but by the end of 1909 adulteration of that sort was rare.[81] The Bureau recorded continued complaints from manufacturers and suppliers that it was impossible to achieve improved quality, but discounted these claims by demonstrating the availablity of unadulterated specimens.[82] Prosecution for adulteration, mislabelling, or substitution was, however, rare in the early years of the act. The Bureau was more concerned to investigate and record than to prosecute, hoping that they would thus be able to influence the behaviour of producers. To some extent this tactic worked, and the manufacturers became increasingly sensitive to the threat of inspection. For example, when one incident occurred involving Smith Kline and French, in which a child died from an apparently dangerous remedy, one of the major concerns of the scientific staff was to avoid an investigation by the Bureau of Chemistry under the 1906 Act.[83] The company was willing to expend considerable energy and money either to defeat the complainant in the local court or to settle rather than to suffer the publicity of an investigation.

If the act led to any tangible achievements in the first years it was to reduce the alcohol and narcotic levels in patent medicines and to standardise state laws.[84] Hand's medicines were all reformulated to remove narcotic contents,[85] and the alcohol in Hofstetter's Bitters declined from 39 per cent to 25 per cent despite falling demand.[86] Both these preparations were sold by large-scale manufacturers.

The first case brought by the government against a drug preparation concerned Harper's CUFORHEDAKE BRANEFUDE.[87] Harper was a Philadelphia College of Pharmacy graduate who had received some laboratory and commercial experience at John Wyeth and Brothers. He left Philadelphia to set up business in Washington around 1890 and sold his medicine as a headache cure. Its main ingredients were alcohol and acetalanid, a synthetic painkiller derived from coal tar and imported from Germany. Though Harper seemed willing to adjust his label after the passage of the act, Wiley was intent on pressing a charge of mislabelling.[88] Extensive debate in court followed, during which the prosecution called in such pharmacologists as Reid Hunt from the Hygienic Laboratory and eminent Washington physicians to testify as to the dangers of acetlanid and the inefficacy of Harper's medicine. The defence, relying on its own expert testimony, showed convincingly that the medicine was not a poison. But the jury was charged only to determine whether the medicine was mislabelled or its packages deceptive. With that instruction the jury could only find Harper guilty of deceptive practices for indicating that the medicine was a 'brain food' of some kind.[89]

Of the first thousand notices of judgement of prosecutions under the 1906 Act, 376 dealt with drugs which had made extravagant claims, contained unidentified compounds, or were adulterated. Included among these were a large number of antibacterial agents, which were used in an attempt to exploit the new prestige of asepsis.[90] In these drugs all disease was associated with germ origins: the drugs were alleged to cure everything from 'blood disorders' (as in the case of septicaemia) to insomnia. Radam's Microbe Killer[91] advertised cures by killing microbes in blood for all diseases: anaeamia, asthma, cancer, consumption, diabetes, diphtheria, grippe, malaria, paralysis, pneumonia, yellow fever. Proscribed by the act, Dr Radam's product was twice seized and his stocks destroyed, but he continued to prosper nevertheless.[92]

Some of the medicines claimed to treat diphtheria effectively. Notice of Judgment 54 dealt with Muco-Solvent which was a specific cure for diphtheria, catarrh, croup, whooping cough, and all throat troubles.[93] Humbug Oil similarly claimed to cure diphtheria. It contained '60% hydro-alcoholic, ammonia, codine, and 40% oils – half turpentine, half linseed.[94] The makers of Humbug Oil were found guilty and given a nominal fine of $5. A main concern at the time was to rid the market of these products rather than jailing or bankrupting the businessmen who produced the medicines.

Large companies with analytical laboratories, however, continued to survive largely unaffected by the legislation. In February 1907, only seven months after the passage of the act, Smith Kline and French published Mahlon Kline's 'Digest of National Food and Drug Act and Regulations'.[95] The following year Willard Graham, of the same company, interpreted the act for manufacturers, defending its value to the public and pointing out that 'only competent and reliable firms [can now be] engaged in the manufacture of Pharmaceuticals'.[96] He described the 'vast amount of analytical work and other labor' necessary and noted that 'over Three Thousand Five Hundred separate analyses have been made in this laboratory to protect ourselves from any violation of the law'.[97]

In a ten-year retrospect on the act, Wiley's successor, Carl L. Alsberg stressed the relationships between the Bureau and the industry. One aspect of the enforcement of the act was to prevent unfair competition. This, he explained, was the reason that the industry was so willing to cooperate.

> Indeed, the Bureau is not infrequently appealed to by the industries to compel the cessation of unfair practices and to encourage the standardization of products when the industry is incapable by itself of bringing about these rules.[98]

In some ways the enforcement acted as a second means of dealing with monopoly and unfair trading practices. The major producers, in any case, saw the act in this light.[99]

Beside the power of the regulation to curb practices which brought discredit to the industry, the new intervention of government was an influence which drew competitors together into associations.[100] The functions of such associations varied from arranging trading agreements to lobbying, but they also aimed to support the technical capabilities of the industry.

> These associations have come to understand the value of constructive work and some of them devote considerable sums annually to experimental research designed to solve the technical problems with which the industry is confronted. Thus, there is made available to the small manufacturer, scientific assistance which would ordinarily be obtainable only by large corporations maintaining their own staff of investigators.[101]

The government approved of these associations. Through close links with such associations, the regulators realised that they could have considerable impact on the industry.

> Since the Bureau of Chemistry has always regarded it as its duty not merely to report violations of the law but also to prevent violations by constructive work intended to improve methods of manufacture, it cooperates actively with such associations of manufacturers. Such cooperation by the various Government agencies is bound to exert the profoundest influence on the country's industrial and social development[102]

The American Pharmaceutical Manufacturers' Association was one group whose organisation was stimulated by the legislation. Led by those same prominent companies which had lobbied for regulation, the association maintained mutually agreeable relations with the government.

The effects of the acts on the drug industry were not limited to business practice. They restricted the entry of small manufacturers and forced existing ones either to expand to the point where they could support a scientific staff, or to merge with larger companies. The significance of legislation and litigation concerning drugs finally hinged on the extent to which the pharmaceutical manufacturers themselves affected the establishment of standards, and whether they could avoid prosecution. Mulford and Smith Kline maintained close contact with the Bureau and had some effect on the standards imposed.[103] Their concern was to set criteria which could not easily be met by competitors. Hence they sought to define which medicines could be considered legitimate cures for a specific disease.[104] Already the leaders assumed that specific cures should be required, an assumption which questioned the legitimacy of all general tonics and panaceas. The companies insisted on a high standard of purity that could not be met by small operations. They could also rely upon the support of the medical community to testify to the efficacy of their scientifically advanced medicines.[105] Even though Mulford and other manufacturers could not hope to take over from patent medicine makers completely, they did gain in prestige as champions of scientific therapeutics by vilifying the so-called quacks. The small manufacturers whom they condemned were not all selling drugs intended to serve as panaceas: many of them claimed to sell scientifically developed, specific remedies. Most of the medicines in fact contained recognised therapeutic agents, such as alcohol, quinine, camphor, and other substances that could be found in pharmacopoeiae.[107]

Enacted early among regulatory activities, the 1902 and 1906 Acts were inconsistently enforced and awkwardly administered. They were implemented by different agencies: control over biologicals were exercised by the Hygienic Laboratory of the Marine Hospital and Public Health Service, while the Pure Food and Drugs Act was executed by the Bureau of Chemistry, Department of Agriculture. Their methods of enforcement differed markedly, with the Bureau of Chemistry relying on complaints and occasional checks, while the Hygienic Laboratory administered licences which specified periodic inspections and the constant monitoring of products from all the producers of biologicals, including foreign companies which exported to the United States.

The relative significance of the two acts has been distorted by historians.[107] Though the 1906 Act was more widely applied, the 1902 Act had a more direct influence over the producers of a limited line of ethical pharmaceuticals and identified the criteria for enforcement, standards and licensing much more clearly and directly. Both acts were supported by major producers in the area but the earlier one provided a real opportunity to specify which producers were working within the guidelines of the law, and which were not. It also provided that violators, or at least those whose products or facilities seemed substandard, could be denied licences and closed down. Both acts encouraged the establishment of large operations of laboratories, inspectors, clerks and administrators to enforce and analyse the products and producers under review, and both establishments conducted research into the basic chemistry, biology and pharmacology of drugs. In so far as the legislation marked a milestone in the development of the drug industry, then, it was to give legal support to the notion of scientific practice, and to rationalise the character of the industry accordingly.

7 The Uses of Science

The variety of ways in which science could be used was well explored by the pharmaceutical companies in the early twentieth century. Technical competence and research capabilities improved at some firms and some new products were developed. Competition with other companies was waged in scientific terms and physicians were addressed in similarly technical language. Medical practitioners were bombarded with advertisements describing new developments, particularly in bacteriology, and were becoming increasingly attuned to the idea of specific causes and remedies. An alliance between drug firms and medicine was being forged in the name of science, and in opposition to proprietary medicines. The implications of this ideology for the companies involved increased quality control, more standardisation of products, a streamlined organisation, and efficient production and marketing techniques.

SCIENCE IN THE DRUG COMPANIES: GENERAL TRENDS

In the drug industry, as in other sectors, the assimilation of scientific personnel and procedures occurred rapidly between the late 1890s and the First World War. Alfred Chandler has characterised this period by some leading examples:

> By the first decade of the new century Western Electric, Westinghouse, General Electric, Electric Storage Battery, McCormick Harvester (and then International Harvester), Corn Products, Du Pont, General Chemical, Goodrich Rubber, Corning Glass, National Carbon, Parke Davis, and E. R. Squibb all had extensive departments where salaried scientifically trained managers and technicians spent their careers improving products and processes. Other companies soon followed suit. The research organizations of modern industry enterprises remained a more powerful force than patent laws in assuring the continued dominance of pioneering mass production firms in concentrated industries.[1]

Pharmaceutical manufacturing was only just beginning to take on the form of a mass-production, concentrated industry of the type exemplified by the electrical manufacturers, but it emerged from the First World War ready to assume that shape. Science played a central role in bringing the industry to this stage.

The most significant change in the character of the industry by 1910 was in company size; although some firms remained very small, the most important, like Mulford and Parke Davis, were growing to considerable proportions. There ensued market battles between large national manufacturers and the smaller, local producers. The tableting machines introduced in the early 1890s allowed the large firms to mass-produce standard preparations, while their rudimentary analytical laboratory procedures permitted them to make new claims about the reliability of their products. Large companies also tended to undercut local producers' markets by selling to a particular constituency – physicians, pharmacists, public health bodies – rather than concentrating on a special region.

There was not only competition between large and small companies, but also between firms within each group. It became particularly fierce between the larger producers, who relied increasingly on novelties, such as new biological medicines, to open new markets and bolster their image as scientifically advanced producers. Although the advertising etiquette of the day discouraged the naming of competitors, contrasting claims were used routinely. Customers were encouraged to 'Ask for Mulford's' or 'Always specify Parke Davis', and such admonitions became regular additions to 'informational' as well as advertising copy. The over-all outcome of these measures to compete more directly both for market sector and national distribution was a slight reduction in the number of firms, a growth in the size of the largest producers, and a widening gap between reputable and less solid companies. The polarisation and rationalisation of the industry was assisted by attempts to force compliance with *Pharmacopoeia* and *National Formulary* standards.

COMPETITION AND THE USE OF SCIENCE

Scientific terminology came to be widely used in promoting products. The benefits of electricity had long been employed in patent medicine advertisements and as early as the 1880s 'microbe killing' was proclaimed as a key attribute of drugs such as Radam's therapy.[2]

During the late 1890s a wide range of scientific qualities, such as specific effect, came to be associated with new drugs and were used in their promotion by the leading companies. A range of acceptable terminology was implicitly established by the end of the century. Drugs could be described, for example, as having been 'tested' or 'standardised'. Advertisements, placed in the medical press and in pamphlets directed at physicians, often cited technical literature, a practice extended by 1900 to include a wide range of English, French and German works. While the producers of biologicals were the first routinely to use extensive technical citations in advertisements for their medicines, the practice soon spread to other sectors.

By examining a few typical companies we can see the variety of other uses of science, as companies began to relate as much to manufacturing processes and laboratory work as to rhetoric. Lederle Laboratories was one that epitomised the science-based companies which were established in the first decade of the twentieth century.

The company was formed by a chemist, Ernst Joseph Lederle, who already had a strong background in bacteriological testing and public health work. He had studied with the chemist, Charles Frederick Chandler, at Columbia College's School of Mines (BA in 1886) and worked in the New York City Health Department, first as a milk inspector and chemist and then, in 1896, as chief chemist after receiving his PhD from Columbia University.[3] The pure milk movement gave Lederle the opportunity to rise within New York city politics and in 1901 he was well placed to be Republican Mayor Seth Low's choice as Health Commissioner and President of the Board of Health. Working from the strong base established in the Board of Health by Herman Biggs and T. Mitchell Prudden, Lederle was able to extend the reformism for which the New York city board had come to stand.

Lederle had been centrally involved with William H. Park in the establishment of the department's pioneering diphtheria antitoxin laboratory. By the time he took office as health commissioner, New York city was one of the largest producers of the antitoxin, public or commercial, and had endured five years of criticism from commercial manufacturers. This criticism was strongest from manufacturers outside New York and focused on the practice of selling to other city health departments. Lederle ended this practice in 1902, ostensibly as a consequence of a petition signed by over a thousand physicians and druggists. His action soon served him well.

When Low's fusion administration lost the election a year later,

Lederle was pushed aside by Tammany Hall. He quickly arranged sufficient capital to incorporate a business for 'chemical, bacteriological and sanitary investigations and analysis'.[4] He took with him, from the Board of Health, Dick Wadsworth and the board's former auditor, Frederic D. Bell. Financial and management help came from his wife's brother, Ronald Taylor, and her brother-in-law, William Larimer Mellon, who headed the Gulf Oil Corporation.[5] Relations with the New York board remained genial, and, since a number of customers continued to request Park's antitoxin after the board stopped distribution, Lederle filled the gap. It proved an enormous advantage to be able to draw upon the former customers of the New York city laboratory. Many had come to trust Park and to expect his preparation. Since this was exactly what Lederle supplied, he unabashedly associated his product with that of his former employer. Most importantly, he could assure other city health departments that the service they would receive would be comparable to that which Park had provided.

With a ready market at hand, Lederle incorporated the Lederle Antitoxin Laboratories as an offshoot of his analytical business. Early in 1906 it received its licence from the US Hygienic Laboratory, the seventeenth such approval for the manufacture of biological products.[6] Unlike any of the other major producers, Lederle entrusted his marketing elsewhere, to Schieffelin and Company, the wholesalers whose director he knew from the Columbia School of Mines.[7] Antitoxin production was commenced in the stables of the New York Veterinary Hospital near the offices of the laboratory. Within a year it moved to what became Lederle's corporate site at Pearl River, New York. Two Yale scientists, Isaac Harris and Stanley D. Beard, were now employed to run the new antitoxin production laboratories.

Lederle himself continued to work for state and city public health departments, acting as consultant sanitary engineer to the New York City Department of Water Supply and on the New York State Water Supply Board. His continuing work in local government led him back to the office of Health Commissioner from 1910 to 1914, and during this time he turned his interests in the laboratories over to another brother-in-law, Matthew Taylor. After his term of office, he returned to his consulting work and served as adviser to the Alien Property Custodian in 1916.

In its first year the Lederle Antitoxin Laboratories filled orders from the boards of health in Chicago[8] and Philadelphia. Philadelphia purchased 2 250 000 units to supplement their distribution requirements.[9] Lederle's scientific staff was from the start more highly skilled (though smaller) than that of most of the commercial competitors, with the exception of Parke Davis and Mulford. In the first years of their employment, the scientists concentrated on maintaining the level of quality Park had reached for the city's antitoxin. Laboratories needed to be assembled, suitable stables erected, and a demanding market supplied. Some members of the staff also found time to publish their related researches. Lederle promoted its antitoxin on the strength of the scientific background of the associated staff; it was the first company to begin antitoxin production on a large scale with an expert staff as its only selling point. This was the kind of competition which the Philadelphia science-based companies now had to face.

The Philadelphia firm, Wyeth Company, aimed less at being science-based than science-associated. It developed a scientific style of rhetoric with little investment in accompanying hardware. It never developed a reputation for scientific research or for introducing new medicines, but it did use advanced tableting machines which allowed it to supply convenient dosages of the most popular preparations. It also presented medical testimonials for its products and accompanied all of its preparations with pamphlets or fliers showing extensive expert support. One such pamphlet from the end of the century was supported by thirty-five citations from German, French and British, as well as American sources.[10] Over one hundred such pamphlets were produced to accompany Wyeth products, all written in a style which was intended to impress through its terminology, but which nevertheless was easily comprehensible to physicians with the most outdated training or to medically informed consumers. Some of these forerunners of package inserts were either written by leading medical figures or were reprints of their work. For example, an early pamphlet[11] which accompanied a digestive powder, was reprinted from the *New York Medical Journal*, written by a prominent New York physician Austin Flint, Jr.

Around 1905 Wyeth began a direct mail campaign 'to physicians only' promoting new products or explaining new expert opinion on the use of a standard preparation such as chromium sulphate.[12] This tactic was sufficiently successful for Wyeth to do a brisk business with the leading chemical companies and drug suppliers of the region. Company records from the first decade of the century show business transactions with Philadelphia's Powers, Weightman and Rosengarten Company and a number of New York manufacturers and suppliers, including McKeeson and Robbins, Merck and Company and Charles Pfizer and Company.[13]

At Smith Kline and French, science took a more active form: the company's laboratories had grown rapidly in the last years of Lyman Kebler's directorship. Though they had remained a service part of the company, their role began to diversify with the addition of new staff. A number of trained assistants were hired in the first decade of the century and the company began to pay increasing attention to the inclusion of skilled and imaginative men in the laboratory. By 1901 Kebler had brought in a pharmacy student, Willard Graham, and Charles D. French, the son of a local chemical manufacturer. In that year he also enticed Joseph England away from Mulford and oversaw C. Mahlon Kline, the son of the company's director, in the laboratory.[14]

C. Mahlon Kline, the son of Mahlon N. Kline, used the laboratory for his apprenticeship in the company, in contrast to the pattern established by the other directors who had worked their way through the marketing departments. His father had earlier seen the importance of scientific training, and Kline was sent to Yale's Sheffield Scientific School.[15] At Yale he studied chemistry under the eminent teachers Professors Russell Chittenden and Lafayette Mendel. He joined Smith Kline and French upon graduation in 1901 and became superintendent of the laboratory for the period 1903 to 1910. Since he was being trained as a manager, he was involved in a variety of other activities beyond the laboratory, and his work as superintendent of the department was shared with others who evidently concerned themselves more exclusively with its daily operation.

Joseph England, the most prominent scientist in the laboratory, was lured from his position in charge of the pharmaceutical department of the H. K. Mulford Company in 1901. He had been the star graduate of the Philadelphia College of Pharmacy in 1883 and had spent sixteen years as chief druggist at the Philadelphia Hospital.[16] England's terms of employment were unique. He was to be paid a salary of $1500 per annum[17] with the provision that he would receive considerably more if his work led to further profits. The company had great expectations of him; they hoped to achieve profitable results from the implementation of his ideas for the Food Department. The Eskay Albumenized Food Products Department had recently been established after experiments made during 1895 and 1896. Marketed primarily as baby and invalid food, the preparation was:

placed in the hands of several physicians who had connections with children's hospitals, or who had opportunity in their private practice to thoroughly test its virtues.[18]

Throughout the later 1890s the company worked on ways to perfect the product, overcoming the difficulties of dissolving albuminoids satisfactorily. By 1910 the Eskay line was a major seller of the company, vigorously promoted through the medical profession.[19] The technical problems with the food line had prompted the company to look for outside aid. They found it in Joseph England:

> In taking up the work please bear in mind that our principal desire in adding you to our force, is to go carefully and thoroughly over our processes and introduce improvements wherever possible, both in the quality of goods, in the methods of manufacture, and in the appearance and finish of the goods.[20]

They offered him a strong incentive to accept the position: in return for working with the food department, England would receive 25 per cent of the net profits of any new specialties he introduced, up to a maximum for salary and commissions of $5000 a year. As his second task, he was to take charge of the pharmaceutical department of the laboratory and 'provide for us formulas for specialties that we could introduce to the medical profession or the community at a profit.[21]

The organisation of Smith Kline and French's departments was such that almost total responsibility for producing and promoting products rested with the groups which manufactured them. The complex arrangement worked out between the laboratory and the food department, for example, included advertising and discounting, profit-sharing and commissions. Advertising was of particular importance. When England originated one of the long-term best sellers, Neurophosphate, the company agreed 'to push the Neuro Phosphates mainly through the agency of the force representing Eskay's Food Department on the road'.[22]

Neurophosphate was developed by England with the assistance of John G. Roberts, an English immigrant, was first employed in Smith Kline's Wine and Oil Department in 1896. Moving to the pharmaceutical department he:

> had the task of filling Hands Chafing Powder with a foot-operated machine that filled and sealed the cans one at a time in a small closed room under a skylight.[23]

He began work in the production laboratory around 1900, where his job was 'to stir a kettle of boiling aqueous solution of opium for three weeks, with a wooden paddle'.[24] Roberts was an exceptionally ambitious young man – a 'tyro' who was not content with such tasks. He studied part-time at the Philadelphia College of Pharmacy and earned his certification in 1905. Shortly after that he was hired by England and set to work in making alkaloidal estimates, a major function within the laboratory. In 1912 he was promoted to become head of the laboratory, despite the claims of a number of other scientists with much greater seniority.

England also employed F. S. McCartney, a graduate from the Pharmacy College in 1892 who pursued further work there before slowly working for an MD at the Medico-Chirurgical College and later at Jefferson Medical College. McCartney had travelled considerably before returning to settle in Philadelphia. He had worked in the drug trade in Pittsburgh and New York and brought with him a variety of promotional techniques. Furthermore, he had studied bacteriology at the Medico-Chirurgical College under Joseph McFarland while the latter was setting up the laboratory for the H. K. Mulford Company. He was clearly a valuable addition to the laboratory.[25]

Further links with major competitors were forged when England hired William Alexander Pearson in 1908. Pearson had a remarkable background which made him a most attractive employee. Trained in chemistry at the Ferris Institute, he earned a PhD in 1902 from the University of Michigan for studies in bacteriology as well as organic and physiological chemistry. Upon graduation he entered Parke Davis's Department of Experimental Medicine, where he had been employed part-time while completing his doctorate.[26] Pearson worked on biological products in Detroit until hired away by H. M. Alexander to work at their Marietta, Pennsylvania, vaccine farm in 1906. In 1908 he was engaged to take charge of Smith Kline and French's analytical department attracted, among other things, by the opportunity to continue academic work at the Hahnemann Medical College in chemistry and toxicology. He later earned an MD after seven years of intermittent study. Pearson's physiological interests were drawn upon when he established a physiological department at Smith Kline and French around 1911.[27] Pharmacodynamics had become particularly important by then due to rising expectations for drug efficacy. In Philadelphia, Mulford had been conducting physiological tests since 1895, and the 1902 Act controlling the production of biologicals stipulated that physiological testing be carried out. Though Smith Kline and French produced no vaccines, physiological testing had become an accepted procedure particularly for assessing and standardising stimulants. Pearson continued to work at the company as a

consultant after taking the post of Professor of Chemistry at Hahnemann in 1912.

The analytical laboratory was already well-equipped by the turn of
the century. There were a number of microscopes, well-stocked
chemical and glass cabinets and, after Pearson arrived, physiological
apparatus and an animal laboratory.[28] From its beginning at 305
Cherry Street, in 1889, it expanded into neighbouring buildings, finally
encompassing much of Cherry Street between Third and Fourth
Streets.[29]

The laboratory performed two main functions: it protected the
company from purchases of inferior raw materials and it standardised
the finished products. In assaying shipments of raw drugs, the chemists
could reject clearly inferior lots, or:

> for example, if a fluid extract is found by assay to be of greater
> potency than the standard, the strength is reduced by adding the
> proper amount of the original menstruum or a former lot which had
> previously been found to be below the standard. Should the assay
> show that the fluid extract was below standard, and no stronger lot
> available, concentration is obtained by evaporation.[30]

Preparations were adjusted to *Pharmacopoeia* standards and, after
1906, kept within the tolerances established by the Pure Food and
Drugs Act. The published results of the laboratory show extreme
variation among the samples, though the range in strength seemed to
vary equally between those too potent and those too diluted, so that in
most cases mixing would result in acceptable solutions.

Discussions of laboratory techniques and reviews of pharmaceutical
problems were occasionally published by members of the laboratory,
usually in the *American Journal of Pharmacy*.[31] Willard Graham
published a variety of results called simply 'Laboratory Notes'.[32] C. M.
Kline demonstrated his scientific acumen soon after arriving at the
laboratory in an article on 'African Balsam of Copaiba'[33] and Joseph
England wrote on 'Tincture of Nux Vomica, 1900', suggesting that the
Pharmacopoeia should revise its formula.[34] George Pancoast published a number of articles of more general interest to pharmacists,
identifying the commercial applicability of certain products and
commenting on sales practices.[35] He wrote in a more informal style
than his other colleagues, addressing the pharmacist as a customer and
discussing sales practices. W. A. Pearson's publications kept him in the
mainstream of academic life.[36] In addition to his contributions to the
American Journal of Pharmacy, which were more complicated than

those of his colleagues,[37] he interpreted such esoteric issues as the standardisation of diphtheria antitoxin for pharmacists,[38] on which he had worked at Parke Davis and at H. M. Alexander.[39] Other types of publications from the laboratory were directed to retailers and covered material which dealt especially with new government practices. These were not research reports and were distributed more widely than typical pharmaceutical publications.

The laboratory operated satisfactorily through the 1920s, enabling the company to project a scientific image, to protect themselves from contaminated or adulterated raw materials, and to standardise and test products. Its existence bolstered Mahlon Kline when he asked Congress in 1906 for stricter standards of quality and purity,[40] as well as allowing the firm to stay within the law after the act was passed without having to change the firm's operation significantly. With the notable exception of England's development of Neurophosphates, the laboratory did not, however, produce many important new products. It did, on the other hand, allow the firm to market drugs which employees such as Pearson and England had produced in other companies.

Smith Kline and French's transformation from a small manufacturing pharmacy to a wholesaler, and thence to a diversified manufacturing and wholesaling operation, paralleled the growth of other expanding businesses in this period. Its sales figures show remarkable growth. In 1886 they had surpassed $700 000 in sales, reaching the one million dollar mark in 1892. Despite the feared effects of competition from Sharp and Dohme, now based in Philadelphia, Smith Kline and French sold $3 million-worth of merchandise in 1902, most of it as proprietary drugs. Its growth through the war was remarkable, and in the post-war economic boom it sold over $7 million-worth of over fifteen hundred products, still mostly non-prescription items.[41]

In the first two decades of the twentieth century, the number of trained scientists, particularly chemists, rose rapidly. Some became teachers and strengthened this trend, but many headed for industry.[42] Most were employed as routine workers, rather than researchers or developers of new techniques and products. For those who entered the drug companies, the work was very similar in form to what they would have undertaken in another industrial sector. Many retained some connection with academic institutions and as a result passed information about the latest studies to their commercial employers.

The large number of such trained personnel was a new resource for the drug companies and they used them and their scientific knowledge in a variety of ways. In a small way, a company like Wyeth used only a limited amount of science, for terminology in its advertisements or for some qualitative and quantitative standardisation to conform to the United States *Pharmacopoeia*. Smith Kline and French employed scientists and their expert knowledge more extensively. Not only did they use it in advertising – even for proprietary medicines – they also standardised in their analytical laboratory in a more routine fashion. They sought to go beyond the legal requirements of the Food and Drugs Act to secure such additional benefits as the identification of inferior goods or the production of reliably regular wares. As the Hand's episode showed, scientific knowledge could also be a useful defence.[43]

Using science on an even larger scale were those companies such as Lederle who could be described as more than just dependent on science, but rather were science-based. Lederle needed its laboratory with its trained scientists to manufacture a bacteriologically sophisticated product upon which it built its business. Little research and development was included in these uses of science. That was restricted to a very few firms, such as Mulford and Parke Davis, and for these, too, it did not figure as the most important responsibility of the scientists they employed.

Joseph England's work might be said to epitomise the use of a scientist – and of science – before the First World War. He oversaw a laboratory that ensured the company a licence; he tested and standardised drugs; he was responsible for some product development; he maintained close relations with the medical community; and he used his scientific expertise to explain his company's products and, when necessary, to defend them in suitably esoteric terms.

8 Scientific Commercialism: Salvarsan and the Dermatological Research Laboratories

The First World War gave American pharmaceutical companies the opportunity to begin scientific research and development in a systematic way. They were now familiar with other uses of science and had developed their own laboratory techniques through the production and standardisation of biologicals. In international terms, however, they fell far behind the German chemical companies in innovation. Moreover, these German companies extensively used patents to monopolise the market for their innovations, even in the United States. The more backward American companies stood little chance of breaking into this market. However, by the beginning of the war, their own skills were sufficiently well developed for them to consider systematic research and development, and the hostilities with Germany temporarily deprived the German companies both of their markets and their patents. A few American companies were able to exploit the opportunity, and prominent among them was the Dermatological Research Laboratory in Philadelphia.

Patents on medicines were considered taboo before the First World War among those American drug manufacturers who were trying to distinguish their 'ethical' or prescription pharmaceuticals from the remedies of proprietary drug makers. Industrial secrecy was a sufficient safeguard, and some companies such as Mulford even went so far as to promote an antimonopolistic stand so as to improve their public relations.[1] Besides, there were few benefits from patenting the insignificant number of advanced drugs developed in American laboratories during the period. Most firms concentrated instead on cultivating new markets and on perfecting the technologies of large-scale production and distribution. The big money-makers which could be monopolised by the ethical pharmaceuticals manufacturers were products such as dietary supplements and baby foods, which relied upon consistent quality and a mass market, or products such as diphtheria antitoxin where the expense of laboratory facilities and a substantial scientific staff necessarily excluded many firms from the market.

German chemical companies, on the other hand, were patenting sophisticated new drugs in large numbers in the United States by 1900.[2] American patent law held no restrictions for foreigners claiming monopoly rights on their developments; there was no requirement even that the products should be manufactured or, indeed, marketed in the United States.[3] This provided the opportunity for German drug companies to take out US patents on any new final or intermediary product developed in their laboratories.[4] By 1905 this procedure had become a carefully devised strategy of patenting every chemical in the course of a research effort, effectively patenting around the final, marketable drug. This technique was successful in discouraging competition because there was little incentive to work through a development phase when patents were already held on every conceivable related product.[5] Used, as it was, as a consistent strategy, it assured German dominance of the American chemical and pharmaceutical market for a number of key products.[6] In the areas of research and marketing they were unchallenged until the First World War threatened their routes to the United States.

GERMAN SALVARSAN IN THE UNITED STATES

Early in January 1917, while the United States was still debating whether to enter the war in Europe, the U-boat *Deutschland* docked in New York harbour with a highly valuable freight including a number of cases of the antisyphilitic drug Salvarsan, or '606'. The *Deutschland* was a cargo submarine designed to run the British blockade so that German industry could continue to export valuable commodities and to bring in some of the critical raw materials the military effort required. In this case the submarine was used to ship Salvarsan in order to support the anxious owner of a subsidiary of a German chemical manufacturer.[7]

Salvarsan had been developed in 1909 by Paul Ehrlich and his associates at Ehrlich's institute in Frankfurt-am-Main, during the now famous search for the 'magic bullet' to treat syphilis. Hoechst routinely patented in the United States developments made in its laboratories and the close ties between Ehrlich's independent institute and the company made cooperation over Salvarsan easy. Between 1898 and 1912 Ehrlich secured about three American patents a year and another half dozen were issued to other Hoechst-sponsored scientists.[8] The American patent for Salvarsan was entrusted to the New York chemical importer and Hoechst representative, the H. A. Metz Laboratories.[9]

Herman A. Metz, president of the laboratories, was a major New York businessman and government official who had been comptroller of the city of New York from 1906 until 1910, a member of the City Board of Education and State Board of Charities, and a representative in the 63rd Congress (from 1913–15) as Democrat from the 10th District in New York.[10] He had extensive interests in chemical manufacturing and importing, dating back to his apprenticeship with the manufacturing druggist Paul Schulze-Berge in Newark. Metz studied chemistry at Cooper Union and then worked his way up in the laboratory of the New Jersey firm.[11] By 1899, when he was 33 years old, Metz had become president and virtual owner of the company. In 1903 it split into H. A. Metz and Company, which concentrated on importing chemicals and dyestuffs, and Victor Koechl and Company, which produced pharmaceuticals. Metz's ties with German chemical manufacturers were secure from the time the firm was owned by Schulze-Berge. The company had acted as agents of Dahl and Company, a dyestuff manufacturer in Bremen, and later of A. Leonhardt and Company near Frankfurt.[12] This arrangement was not atypical, as the other major German chemical companies, including the Big Six which later created the Dye Monopoly, all either formed American subsidiaries or consigned their markets to American representatives. One of the more important tasks of these American businesses was to protect the German patent-holder.

For example, Badische (BASF) was represented by Messrs William Pickhardt and Kuttroff, who were the successors to the Badische Company in America.[13] The Bayer Company was represented by E. Sehlback and Company, who were later succeeded by the Farbenfabriken of Elberfeld Company, and then by the American Bayer Company. These importers and representatives were all in New York and their responsibilities ranged from marketing to maintaining patents.[14]

The Farbwerke Hoechst (Meister, Lucius and Bruning) had been represented by American agents since the 1880s. In 1890 they contracted the responsibility for this to the firm for which Metz worked. The Hoechst account was very important, Metz later recalled, because antipyrin, the first of the important coal-tar medicinals, was controlled by the German company. Moreover:

> With the Hoechst account, the firm also secured the control of lanolin, then controlled by a United States patent, and the sale of the products of I. B. Ibels of Brussels, a small but efficient maker of certain colors, such as magenta, phosphine, nigronine, etc., used largely for leather.[15]

By 1910 Metz had firm control of Hoechst products in the United States, and thus he controlled Ehrlich's Salvarsan patent as well. But by the time the *Deutschland* had docked in New York, Metz faced a serious challenge to the monopoly which had been entrusted to him.[16] Salvarsan was now a well-accepted therapy for syphilis. Scarcity of the drug, due to the British blockade of Germany, therefore created great consternation both among physicians, who had already started patients on Salvarsan treatment, and among pharmacists, who wished to respond to the growing demand for the drug. The uproar in 1917 over the inaccessibility of Salvarsan followed seven years of controversy over the effectiveness of the drug and its proper use. In the United States in particular the response ranged from uncritical acceptance to xenophobic resistance.[17]

Clinical testimonials both favourable and critical had begun shortly after Ehrlich's publication of his results, and proliferated after 1911 when test samples were made available.[18] During these first years, all trials were conducted with small experimental lots supplied directly from Ehrlich's Frankfurt laboratory, having been tested at the Georg Speyer Haus, the research facility Ehrlich established in 1906 with funds from a local philanthropist.[19] In addition to an eagerness on the part of many American clinicians to try the remedy, the popular press fastened on to the subject of the magic bullet and the lay community began to discuss both syphilis and its treatment in a newly open manner.[20] This led to a vigorous effort on the part of physicians to investigate the drug, and encouraged syphilis patients to request Salvarsan treatment. As the techniques for administering Salvarsan became more refined and the expectations of cure more widely understood, the American medical community came to rely upon the drug. Despite this widespread interest there was a marked lack of research, however, because of the patent barricade Hoechst had so effectively constructed.

AMERICAN SALVARSAN

The first infringement in the Salvarsan patent occurred in Philadelphia in 1916, after the Dermatological Research Laboratories (DRL) finally synthesised the drug.[21] The DRL was organised as a non-profit institution in 1912 by Drs Jay Frank Schamberg, John A. Kolmer and George W. Raiziss to study psoriasis, a metabolic disorder which causes flaking and scaling of the skin.[22] The director, Schamberg, was an upright, meticulous man with a strong sense of academic purpose and clinical mission.[23] His position as professor in the prominent University of Pennsylvania Dermatology Department had further increased his stature as the pre-eminent Philadelphia dermatologist. After receiving his MD from the University of Pennsylvania in 1892, he had studied in Europe for a year. Schamberg's prominence was important not only in helping him to secure funds for the establishment of the DRL but, more importantly, for assembling a talented staff for the definition of critical research programmes.[24]

The first men he brought to the laboratories were two other professors from the University of Pennsylvania. Like Schamberg, John A. Kolmer and George W. Raiziss, had been trained in research medicine.[25] Kolmer had a background in pathology and was at the time working in the new area of immunology. Raiziss had been trained in chemistry and was trying to keep at the research front of the quickly evolving area of biochemistry. Like other American medical scientists, Kolmer and Raiziss were faced with grave difficulties in finding support for their research.[26] The medical schools still considered their professors to be part-time teachers rather than researchers. At the University of Pennsylvania, as elsewhere, scientific research was conducted on shoe-string budgets with little support from the medical schools.[27] One strategy medical staff could pursue in seeking a funded laboratory was to establish an institute largely independent of the university. In the case of the Dermatological Research Laboratories, initial funding came from the Philadelphia financier, Peter A. B. Widener, who endowed the institute in 1912. His gift allowed the DRL to be opened in April 1912 in the basement of the hospital of the Philadelphia Polyclinic College for Graduates in Medicine, a post-graduate medical school and hospital later absorbed into the University of Pennsylvania's School of Medicine.[28]

In 1912 Widener had gone to Schamberg suffering from psoriasis.[29] Schamberg explained to Widener that very little was known about the condition. In the course of treatment, Schamberg convinced him to fund the laboratories. Widener had acquired a reputation for penuriousness, especially with regard to medical charity, an area in which Philadelphia philanthropists were expected to be benevolent.[30] This gift dramatically changed his standing.

The results of the major work from the laboratories were published the following year and became classics in dermatology.[31] They consisted of two broad lines of inquiry, one from the bacteriological and pathological point of view, and the other from that of physiology and chemistry. Schamberg and Kolmer believed that some aspects of syphilis therapy might be useful when applied to psoriasis.[32] The first paper, for example, analysed the utility of the Wasserman reaction in establishing a prognosis for psoriasis. In addition to the published papers, the staff at the DRL worked to develop therapies for psoriasis and to test them at the Polyclinic. Around 1914 the group began manufacturing a vaccine made from the various organisms found on psoriasis patients' skin, but this resulted in no improvement when used to treat other patients, or even, in most instances, the same ones.[33]

Although the vaccine was unsuccessful, Schamberg produced a variety of mercury and iodine treatments for psoriasis and made preliminary inquiries into the possibilities of marketing these medicines.[34] In general, the principals thought of the laboratories as an institution concerned with research in chemotherapy and they tried to generalise their psoriasis work as much as possible, especially in the area of therapeutics. In the course of early investigations the staff produced a number of mercurial compounds, one of which, marketed under the name of Mercurophen, came into wide use as an antiseptic.[35]

In 1915 Schamberg, predicting that the British blockade would make supplies from Germany difficult to obtain, set Raiziss to synthesise Salvarsan and its successor, Neosalvarsan.[36] At the outset the difficulty of this task was not appreciated because it was assumed that the patent Paul Ehrlich had taken out in the United States in 1910 would provide sufficient information to synthesise the drug.[37] In fact the complexity of the laboratory procedure, and the need for the know-how possessed only by Ehrlich and his collaborators, at first thwarted Raiziss.[38] After several months of frustrating attempts, however, his efforts eventually yielded the yellow powder, and he began testing its toxicity. His success marked the first production of the drug outside of Germany, although it was soon synthesised in England, France, Japan and Canada.[39] Along with the triumph of Salvarsan's synthesis, however, came the legal problems of patent infringement.[40]

Hermann Metz feared that the combination of anti-German sentiment in America allied with arguments for a moral obligation to allow the product to be sold would make his efforts to block the marketing of the drug by others ineffective. The ethical and legal arguments became particularly strong after the DRL enlisted the support of the medical community.[41] But Metz's strongest argument against the DRL was that Schamberg was motivated neither by ethical considerations nor by scientific curiosity. In later Congressional testimony, he claimed that the Dermatological Research Laboratories 'took up a study of Salvarsan and began to make it when it became scarce'.[42] A narrow legal case for patent infringement could have been clinched on these grounds, as long as Metz proved that the DRL sold the medicine.

TRADE AGREEMENTS

Schamberg's efforts to secure manufacturing rights for Salvarsan began shortly after Raiziss managed to synthesise the drug. At the 1915 annual meeting of the Medical Society of the State of Pennsylvania, Schamberg presented his case to the house of delegates.[43] He was successful in sponsoring a resolution which provided that the Society would urge the Secretary of the Interior or the Commissioner of Patents:

to call upon the patentees of Salvarsan to supply this drug or permit the same to be supplied by others, or to take such other means as his judgement may dictate to relieve the existing condition.[44]

However, this early effort was not successful in forcing Metz to relinquish the patent rights. It became clear that the legal protection of German-held patents had to be challenged first.

Nothing further was done for another year and a half, during which Schamberg continued to manufacture and supply Salvarsan to his regular customers and even to Metz himself. In March of 1917 he renewed his effort to evade the Hoechst patent officially and lobbied Congress to achieve this. He enlisted the medical profession by means of a public petition circulated from the Mayo Clinic addressed to

Franklin H. Martin of the American College of Surgeons. In an accompanying letter, Dr John H. Stokes, a supporter of Schamberg, spelled out the problem.[45] He began with a description of the supply and cost of Salvarsan from before the war. He detailed the price jump from the original set rate of $3.60 per maximum dose to a speculative level of roughly three times that amount, occasionally rising as high as $16 a dose.[46] Metz had entered into an agreement with Schamberg that the DRL could produce Salvarsan for sale to Metz, with the condition, set by Schamberg, that the price be lowered to $2.50 a dose.[47] After Metz received further shipments late in 1915, Hoechst once again took control of the pricing and the cost rose to $4.50 a dose.[48] Stokes claimed that:

> The advance in price and the difficulty of securing the preparations of course still further restricted the use in this country of one of the most important curative agents in existence.
>
> Finally, as a result of the complete suspension of imports, the entire supply of both Neo-salvarsan and Salvarsan in this country failed entirely, and a large proportion of the profession was obliged to return to the antiquated methods in use in pre-Salvarsan days, and to conduct the treatment of syphilis with mercury alone, a slower and less effective procedure, making abortive cure out of the question, and admittedly unsatisfactory in controlling syphilis as a contagious disease.[49]

Since Metz was caught with no stock in the midst of anti-German sentiment, Schamberg was then able to negotiate a second agreement to produce and sell the drug directly.[50] Schamberg's name for this domestic Salvarsan was 'Arsenobenzol' which he succeeded in having entered into the *United States Pharmacopoeia*, with the biological specifications he set at the Dermatological Research Laboratories.[51] Its distribution was allowed by Metz on the understanding that as soon as Hoechst America could re-import, the manufacture of Arseno-benzol would be suspended.[52] In the meantime, Schamberg, Kolmer and Raiziss took every opportunity to publish on the production, use and clinical results of the drug, and built a reputation as the leading American experts on modern syphilis treatment.[53] They also endeavoured to show the superiority of their product over that produced in Germany.[54] This claim was based on the relative effectiveness and low toxicity of the drug, arguments which were not entirely convincing given the somewhat weak experimental results which they and the United States Health Service Hygienic Laboratory published.[55]

During the nine-month period from November 1915 to July 1916 when the DRL was the sole source for Salvarsan, some 25 000 doses of Arsenobenzol were sold.[56] German Salvarsan again became available in July as a result of further trade negotiations and the cost rose from the DRL's price of around $3 up to $4.50.[58] At this time, and up to the rupture of diplomatic relations with Germany, most of the shipments arrived via the *Deutschland*. Stokes asked Congress to consider the alternative to allowing the DRL to sell Salvarsan:

I might mention at this point that the manufacture of arsenical compounds practically identical with Salvarsan has been carried on in the belligerent countries since the beginning of the war. Kharsivan is, I think, the name of the British product, manufactured by the Burroughs Wellcome Company. Diarsenol and Neo-diarsenol are manufactured at Toronto under the direction of the Canadian Government by the Synthetic Drug Company Limited, the direct supervision being carried out by the Medical Department of the University of Toronto. A good deal of the former drug has been used in this country, although its importation is an infringement of the German patents. Reports of its unstable character have appeared in the literature, and I have myself within a short time, nearly had disastrous results in five cases on a single day, from the use of this product, and have known of other serious effects. In view of the fact that its importation is a violation of the patent law, and that it is an unstable and apparently dangerous substitute, it can scarcely be looked upon as a source of supply in an emergency.

Realizing this situation, and believing that the state of our relations with Germany affords the psychological and practical opportunity for terminating this unreasonable monopoly, a number of us have sounded Professor Schamberg on his willingness to place his facilities at the disposal of the government and the medical profession of this country. . . . Suitable action, apparently in the form of an abrogation of these patents by Congress, will make possible the radical reductions in price so much to be desired in the interest of public health. . . . I understand that the German patentees have endeavored to carry through an arrangement with him which will enable him to make Salversan for them, but will maintain the price far above the figure at which he could place it on the market. From such an arrangement he has endeavored to hold back in the effort to accomplish a radical readjustment. I would respectfully urge that governmental action in this matter should be prompt or it will be ineffectual, and relief from the existing unjust state of affairs will be delayed at least eleven years.[58]

PRODUCTION

In June 1917, after the US entered the war and after extensive lobbying by Schamberg, the Senate Committee on Patents finally met to consider a bill 'suspending during the present emergency all rights arising out of any patent granted by the United States upon any compound or medicine of which Salvarsan is a constituent part'.[59] and another bill:

authorizing and directing the Secretary of War or the Secretary of the Navy to manufacture for the use of the Army, Navy or the people of the United States, any drug, medicine, or other remedy or device which is protected by a patent or patents, trade-mark or trade-marks, and which can be procured at a reasonable price within the United States.[60]

The debate which followed between Metz and the supporters of Schamberg was heated and, in the end, unconvincing for either side.[61] Schamberg was represented by Dr George Walker, who also spoke in his official capacity as a professor at Johns Hopkins University. He explained the stand of the DRL in two ways. First he pointed out that the Hoechst monopoly was sufficiently effective to allow Metz to exploit the market whenever he could or wished, and that the price fluctuated wildly at two or three times the previously established cost. Secondly, Walker made an eloquent plea for ethical considerations:

Gentlemen, this is not technical law. This is a question of property rights, this is not somebody's contract; this is a question of saving Americans, children who are infected with syphilis, and it is up to us; it is up to the United States Government to get us out of it in some way or other.

I do not know whether this thing can be abrogated or not, but it is a question where a property right where a contract stands against the interest of the American people, women and children who have been innocently infected and who can not get the drug and who are being turned away every day of the year from hospitals all over the country because we can not get rid of it.[62]

Walker then presented a plan showing how the DRL could supply the drug during the first year after the abrogation of the patent for $2 a dose, in the second year for half that price and from the third year for 50 cents a dose.

There were two immediate responses to Walker's effort. In the next issue of the *Journal of the American Medical Association*, Franklin Martin wrote an editorial supporting the abrogation of the German patent,[63] and Herman Metz issued a rejoinder in a flier addressed 'To the Medical Profession'.[64] Metz admitted that he had a problem of supply, and outlined an arrangement with the DRL to supply Salvarsan to him for distribution. Furthermore, he dropped the price from $4.50 to $2.50 per dose 'to make the product available for the treatment of charity patients and other hospital cases'.[65] Metz then wrote:

> I also call attention again to the fact that Diarsenol and other substitutes for Salvarsan and Neosalvarsan that are being sold are infringements of the rights of the patentees and that all violations of these rights will be prosecuted under the law.[66]

But Metz was losing ground: although the hearings did not immediately lead to the abrogation of the patent, they did so eventually by stimulating physicians to petition Congress. Finally, after a few hearings in various committees,[67] the administration prepared the Adamson Bill which, among other things, authorised the President of the United States to license citizens to operate enemy patents.[68] The Dermatological Research Laboratories was the first business to be licensed.[69] As a result of this they won the contract to supply the military forces with all their Salvarsan during the war and were able to build a huge production facility which proved extremely profitable after the war.[70]

Salvarsan was not the only medicine to be affected by the 1916 cut in supplies. Of the 592 drugs listed in the 1916 edition of *New and Non-Official Remedies*, 228 were imported into the United States from Germany.[71] Among these were Salvarsan and Neosalvarsan, Aspirin, Anesthesine (benzocaine), Veronal (barbitol) and Novocaine. There were no laboratories in the United States attempting to develop drugs along these lines. Even after the war the Chemical Foundation bemoaned the lack of indigenous chemotherapeutic research:

> While there are in the United States a number of institutes and foundations for medical research doing most valuable work, there is none (except for the Dermatological Research Laboratories) in

which the problems are being approached primarily from the chemical standpoint. Consequently, few new lines of chemical investigation in relation to diseases have been developed in this country and we have been largely dependent upon foreign countries, especially Germany, for discoveries relating to the applications of chemistry to disease.[72]

RESEARCH AND COMMERCIALISM

From the outset, Schamberg, Raiziss and Kolmer intended to provide the antisyphilitic to their patients, to the Polyclinic and to other area hospitals.[73] The marketing of Salvarsan by the DRL followed the pattern set by other leading, scientifically oriented pharmaceutical manufacturers.[74] They were especially influenced by their Philadelphia neighbour, the H. K. Mulford Company. Considering their widely contrasting origins, the similarity between the Mulford Company in, say, 1914 with the DRL ten years later is remarkable. Mulford published a technical journal modelled almost exactly after a leading clinical journal, the *Medical Record*, in which the company's laboratory staff presented research results and reprinted clinical reports using Mulford products, or of relevance to biologicals production and treatment.[76] In 1923 the DRL began publishing a journal similar in many ways to the *Mulford Digest*. *Progress in Chemotherapy and Treatment of Syphilis* included research reports from the laboratories, summaries of therapeutic practices or clinical trials using DRL products, and descriptions of scientific procedures at the laboratories.[76]

Even before this, the marketing practices of the DRL had incurred the ire of Herman Metz. In his Senate testimony he claimed that, although the DRL was ostensibly a non-profit organization, it conducted itself in the manner of a competitive enterprise: 'they have salesmen out, and they do business in the regular way, just like anybody else does'.[77] Metz was particularly concerned that the DRL was 'getting away' without paying taxes. This he considered unfair competition as it alone accounted for a profit of $500 000 in 1918, he claimed.[78] Schamberg responded indignantly to such claims:

> Indeed, innuendoes of [commercialism] have from time to time come to our ears, uttered by misinformed or cynical persons, or by those with sordid commercial motives.[79]

Needless to say, he rejected them entirely.

In his attempt to show the DRL to be an operation like his own, Metz did more than point to its commercial aspect. He claimed that his was just as socially beneficial an institution because it too sponsored scientific research.[80] From August 1917 Metz did in fact run a laboratory with at least one MD and one PhD on his staff at all times.

The scientific activities of H. A. Metz Laboratories were guided by Herman's brother, Gustave P. Metz.[81] Gustave had also studied chemistry at Cooper Union (BA in 1896) but unlike his brother continued his studies by attending the Swiss Federal Polytechnic in Zurich and earning a doctorate from the University of Basel in 1902. His brother placed him at Hoechst as a consultant until 1917 when he returned to New York to become vice-president and production manager in Herman's laboratory. There he joined H. Sheridan Baketel, MD, a very well-connected physician who had worked for many years in New York as a general practitioner and medical journalist.[82] Baketel had also been employed as advertising manager for the Denver Chemical Manufacturing Company before joining Metz in 1911 as medical director. By 1917, then, the company had three very important areas covered. Herman, with his business experience and political influence, was a capable director. His younger brother's chemistry training and experience at Hoechst gave the company production know-how, and Baketel managed affairs with the medical community while drawing widely upon contacts there and in the medical press.[83]

One element was missing. The company had no research staff until 1920, despite their need to show that they were contributing to medical knowledge. To rectify this, Metz went to Columbia University's College of Physicians and Surgeons where he arranged to fund laboratory studies by the biochemists Casimir Funk and Augustus Levy.[84] There was, of course, quite a difference between the research staff which the DRL maintained and the supplementary financing Metz offered Funk and Levy. In fact, the only services Metz ever demanded from Columbia were occasional quality checks.[85] However, Metz's accusations of DRL commercialism were soon confirmed.

Military contracts had boosted the fortunes of pharmaceutical companies generally. By the end of the war many of them had considerable amounts of ready money on which they could capitalise.[86] The DRL also came out of the war with an embarrassment of riches, despite the exhaustion of the Widener Trust in 1916. It had accumulated $750 000 as tax-free earnings for the institute.[87]

These profits[88] were something of a burden for the laboratory and, in March 1921, Schamberg resolved his problems by turning over half a million dollars in accumulated profits to a newly-established Dermatological Research Institute and reluctantly prepared the laboratories for sale.[89] The government refused to license the DRL after the end of the war because of its supposed research status. As Schamberg put it:

> Republics are notoriously ungrateful, and the fact that we sold the government Salvarsan at one half the price we could have legitimately charged them, and moreover at a time when they could have got it nowhere else, is either soon forgot or else never known by the general public. In our hearts we are satisfied that we have carried on in the best interests of our country and of the people's health. We have gained nothing personally from the rewards of our work. The war has ended between nations, but the war against disease must go on, and it is for this purpose that we have dedicated our efforts and financial rewards.[90]

The institute, he said, would use all profits from the sales of Arsphenamine and other drugs for further research.[91]

In establishing the institute, Schamberg allowed the word to be circulated that he had finished with the manufacturing aspect of the business and would sell the Salvarsan-producing facility.[92] Metz was of course the obvious purchaser and he reportedly was 'trumpeting that he was prepared to offer $50,000 more than the nearest bidder.'[93] However, in July 1922, representatives from Abbott Laboratories met with Dr Schamberg and expressed an interest in purchasing the plant.[94] Abbott, a medium-sized firm from north Chicago, was interested in expanding with the wealth it had acquired during the war.[95] The first inquiry did not lead to a sale and news that the DRL was still available continued to spread. Later that summer:

> during the lull in the convention of the American Pharmaceutical Manufacturers Association in New York City, Dr Burdick (of Abbott) was playing golf . . . when he heard from William Buffum, an official of the Chemical Foundation that a deal was on a verge of being closed with Metz's representatives. The two hurried to Philadelphia and confronted Dr Schamberg.[96]

'It's not true', he told them, 'I'm not interested in selling to Metz. I don't like the affiliations with Germany' – an understatement summarising many years of conflict with Metz.[97] Negotiations with Abbott continued into September when the selling price of $150 000 for the plant and $31 000 for all stock was agreed upon.[98] It is not easy to assess the appropriateness of this deal. In addition to the physical facilities and Dr Raiziss, who stayed with the manufacturing plant, Abbott acquired the reputable name of the DRL which had waged the 'good fight' against the 'German' Metz and was associated with the academic connections and scholarly standards of the DRL staff.[99]

Those working in the former laboratories divided into two groups, one of which went with Abbott and one of which joined the organisation that Schamberg then renamed as the Research Institute of Cutaneous Medicine.[100] Among the former group were the production experts and salesmen, as well as the manager, Raymond E. Horn, the former confidential secretary to George Wickersham, Attorney-General in the Taft administration. Horn's political contacts had proved valuable to Schamberg and were well appreciated at Abbott.[101]

Metz made one final effort to re-establish his former monopoly by engaging in a price war as soon as Abbott acquired the Salvarsan production plant. Abbott would have had to cut their prices in half to compete directly with Metz, but chose instead to concentrate harder on selling Salvarsan and Neo-salvarsan as treatments for a variety of diseases.[102] As prices stabilised Dr Burdick wrote to Mrs Abbott (the majority stockholder):

> The purchase of the Dermatological Research Laboratories was an exceedingly fortunate venture. This business is not seasonal, it runs about the same throughout the year, with some slight relaxation during the summer months. I think it is perfectly safe to say that we will make during the first year of operation enough to pay for the entire plant.[103]

Although the figures for Abbott's profits from Salvarsan alone are not available, the autumn 1923 figures show sales of $2 154 000, an increase of $503 000 over 1922. The $181 000 purchase price for the DLR had been amply repaid.[104]

The relationship between commercial advantage and the rate and direction of research is clearly evident in this case study. Schamberg and his colleagues at the DRL became acutely aware in 1915 that the production of Mercurophen and other marketable drugs was highly profitable, and that chemotherapy had become one of medicine's most exciting research sites. Whatever image Schamberg might have wished to portray for the DRL, it had become a pharmaceutical manufacturer. The parallels which Herman Metz could see between his operation and Schamberg's lay in their commercial similarity. The difference which Schamberg wished to stress – that the DRL was a reasearch institute – was important, but not in the way he intended it to be understood. Metz's involvement in research might have been a 'front' to gain respectability, but the DRL's active involvement in research did not render it commercially neutral. This very difference between them was rather an indication of the new style now operating amongst the pharmaceutical manufacturers. Substantial research was now being undertaken by a new type of pharmaceutical manufacturer, just as it was in the electrical, chemical and engineering industries.

With its sophisticated research facilities, the DRL was able to synthesise Salvarsan and, hence, to enter a market otherwise monopolised by German chemical companies. The war enabled the laboratories to break the German stranglehold, but although the DRL seemed successfully launched as both a research and a commercial enterprise, its former status as an academic institute did not allow this combination to continue. However, by the early 1920s, other American companies had managed to weld commercialism to sophisticated reasearch facilities and were able to follow the DRL's lead. American pharmaceutical firms such as Abbott Laboratories now undertook a systematic programme of scientific research and development.

9 Modern Medical Manufacturing, 1918–29

THE INDUSTRY TO 1918

Drug makers had evolved from the small manufacturing pharmacies of the 1820s to larger production units with regional markets by mid-century. By investing capital, first in expanded ranges of products and later in more efficient manufacturing techniques, some companies were able to grow to a moderately large size. Army purchases at the beginning of the Civil War and expanded markets after the war allowed enterprising firms to become sufficiently sizeable to take advantage of the opportunities provided by faster transportation and the increased circulation of newspapers. Formal, hierarchical management structures supported this growth by the 1890s. As the medical profession became increasingly science-oriented, so companies too began to consider the possibilities of science. Technical interpretations were increasingly used as drug manufacturers expanded and from before the turn of the century served a number of functions from advertising rhetoric to standardisation. Gradually, company science shifted from merely a veneer to the employment of trained medical scientists.

By the 1890s a few companies began to use such scientifically trained staff for more than product promotion, testing or liaison with the medical community: they began to be used for product development. The production of biological medicines epitomised this new role. The 1902 Biologicals Control Act secured the new position of the scientists, since licences were only granted to firms with a scientific staff and laboratory. Many of these staffs still focused on routine quality control and promotion until the First World War, when product development became increasingly important. The Dermatological Research Laboratory's production of Salvarsan indicated the new direction of American pharmaceutical manufacturing.

We have explored the role of science in bringing the industry to its 1918 form. Other themes in the development of medical manufacturing can now be explored. Competition, for example, provided an impetus to innovation. For most producers this meant recreating an important medicine made by a competitor.[1] Sometimes this would be initiated by consumers who would ask, for instance, why Wyeth was not offering a product similar to one marketed by Smith Kline. The nature of competition in the drug industry changed over the forty years under study. Price competition became less important. This was partly because prices on similar goods more or less stabilised between 1900 and 1920, but also because consumers acknowledged differences in reputation and, to some extent, quality among competitors.[2] Competition through the laboratory formed another stimulus to innovation. New medicines sold better than old medicines and it was the laboratories which were expected to provide such novelties. In some cases, *anything* new would be sufficient. Combination drugs were particularly popular during the 1920s and it took relatively little effort to devise a useful amalgam of standard preparations to combine, for example, a temperature-reducing drug with a stomach-soothing agent.[3]

The drug industry was a science-based industry made up of small businesses, moulded by incentives which the business climate provided and by the action of individual entrepreneurs. The two main routes to the establishment of ethical pharmaceuticals firms were through an expansion of a compounding pharmacy business, and the production of patent medicines. In the case of a large manufacturer/wholesaler like Smith Kline and French, it expanded from a local pharmacy to brand-name packaging and then to large-scale wholesaling. During this early period there were many such small businesses which expanded in this manner. The critical factors in their success seemed to be, first, the ability of the small producer to cultivate a loyal clientele in the medical profession as well as the general public and, then, access to good transportation. The qualities of individual entrepreneurs were significant for the first of these but not for the more important second point. Like the most significant factor in the accumulation of great wealth, place was more important than individual qualities.[4] Philadelphia, as explained in Chapter 2, was a prime location because of its well-developed medical community and excellent trading links with western and southern markets.

The activities of corporate entrepreneurs in the twentieth century took on a different form. In the case of the Mulford Company both personal and corporate entrepreneurial activity were important. Henry Mulford was a classic case of an enterprising person. His talents and interests, however, did not extend far beyond establishing his company and guiding it towards drug research and development. But even in the earliest days of the independent company, Mulford realised that Milton Campbell would be a better administrator than he was and allowed Campbell to take over the entire management of the growing firm. Campbell, though not a trained administrator, devoted himself full-time to that task, leaving Henry Mulford to the technical work of manufacturing pharmacy and hiring departmental directors to organise their special areas.

John Wyeth showed his entrepreneurship in a different way. His business was built on new tableting machines, which gave the Wyeth Company the competitive advantage of larger-scale production. Wyeth could manage the compounding, production and sales of his small company sufficiently well, and seems to have had little incentive to expand the firm to a size larger than he alone could handle. Wyeth also had no desire to create a company dynasty or even to perpetuate it, as he gave his company's assets to Harvard University upon his death. Furthermore, he kept with his one innovation, the mass-production tableting machinery, and made few attempts to innovate further.

The typical characteristic of those companies which led in innovation was the mobility of their staff. These firms – Mulford, Smith Kline and Parke Davis being the most prominent – hired from each other and sought talented scientists from other companies. The leading companies hired men who could bring ideas and, more importantly, techniques from their competitors. There was no sense of company loyalty among medical scientists and they eagerly looked for better offers from other companies. Many scientists moved between at least two companies. This mobility was particularly important in the first fifteen years of the antitoxin era when technical knowledge was vital to the production of biologicals. Parke Davis and Mulford scientists were in great demand and easily moved between the two, or, as in the cases of Lyman Kebler and Joseph England, from one of the leaders to a company wishing to employ a man with particular expertise. Staff mobility became a key to innovation. During this early period the technical literature was inadequate to demonstrate how to duplicate antitoxin or other sophisticated new drugs. Often there were significant omissions, or some subtlety of procedure was not adequately explained.[5] Hence McFarland was hired by Parke Davis after he had set up America's most effective commercial antitoxin-producing laboratory at Mulford.

POST-WAR INDUSTRY

In general the pharmaceutical industry emerged from the First World War stronger than before.[6] Large government contracts, like Mulford's antitoxin arrangement with the army and the Dermatological Research Laboratories' negotiations to provide Salvarsan, gave the companies sufficient funds to make long-term plans.[7] The experience gained from the patent disputes stimulated many companies to begin taking out patents regularly from the mid-1920s.[8] The government's role, though still not settled, was gradually taking shape in the form of effective enforcement of the 1902 Biologicals Control Act against small vaccine producers and enforcement of the 1906 Pure Food and Drugs Act against particularly blatant violators among the patent medicine makers.[9]

The drug industry in the inter-war period was characterised by growth in all sectors and increased market security for ethical pharmaceutical makers. Corporate forms had generally taken shape in most industries before the war, but for pharmaceutical companies, as for other science-based manufacturers, there were a number of basic problems which lingered on to be resolved in the 1920s. The value of research had been demonstrated by a number of leading firms, but laboratories for product development did not become widespread until after the war. Similarly, the continuing task of educating their consumers now settled into an established pattern. Another factor which set a modern pattern for the industry was a series of mergers and take-overs. These solidified the leadership of the industry and placed at the forefront most of the companies which were to become household names. Both amongst the corporations and in the medical community, the role of the drug industry became established during the 1920s on foundations laid in the preceding three decades.

The acquisition of the Dermatological Research Laboratories by Abbott Laboratories in 1922 was the first of the major mergers among small, academically advanced drug makers in Philadelphia.[10] It brought together a growing mid-western drug house, which had a great deal of money available after the war,[11] with a small commercial research group which had led the development of chemotherapeutics in the United Sates. The DRL had shown that the development of a science-based drug was both feasible and profitable, and that

American firms could break the German monopoly of advanced products. It also established a pattern of systematic research and development which could be used elsewhere.

Just as twenty-five years previously the antitoxins had seemed to promise cures for all infectious and contagious diseases, now a wide range of medicines seemed promised by synthetic organic chemistry. Salvarsan was presented as the first in a line of new specific remedies, all based on the side-chain theory of chemical affinities. It seemed that others could be developed using a combination of empirical trial and the increasingly sophisticated tools of organic chemistry. In theory the method was similar to that involved in producing a new biological medicine. The disease would be isolated, either as a toxin in the case of serum therapy, or as a pathogen in the cases of diseases such as syphilis. Then the chemical with the proper affinity for the exuded toxifier could be found through a painstaking matching process. This was similar to the process by which toxin was injected into animals which would produce the proper antibody in their blood serum which could then be extracted and used to cure afflicted humans. The theoretical straightforwardness of both techniques, despite their technical difficulties, were great inducements for potential producers to attempt the manufacture of new medicines.

With drug makers expanding into ever more highly theoretical areas like chemotherapeutics, physicians increasingly relied on them to provide information. The educational function which companies like Mulford and the Dermatological Research Laboratory assumed before and during the war become the acceptable and expected function of drug makers during the 1920s. Although physicians began to look more critically at the information they were receiving, they were also resigned to the fact that only the scientists within the companies and physicians who had conducted clinical tests for the manufacturers had full information about a new product. Within a few months after the introduction of a new product the medical journals might begin to have independent results to publish, but this was not always the case and the results were often far less complete or conclusive than company-provided information.

RELATIONS WITH THE MEDICAL COMMUNITY

With the companies well established as the makers of advanced drugs and the suppliers of the most recent information, their relationship with the medical community grew closer than ever before. Changes within the medical profession itself, however, had a significant impact on the industry.

Alterations in professional allegiances and the rise of specialisation led the way. The AMA had peaked in the percentage of the profession it represented before the war.[12] Its power, though more organised, had become less representative. New organisations representing specialty clinical practices or scientific interests grew. One such association was the American Society for Pharmacology and Experimental Therapeutics.[13] This association was highly sensitive about its members working for the drug companies, as it felt undermined by the bad reputation which indiscriminate endorsements by medical scientists had given the discipline.[14]

The medical schools reflected these changes. The growing influence of scientific medicine was soon felt in the schools.[15] Pharmacology became a more commonly taught area, increasingly presented in the style of organic chemistry rather than the materia medica of the nineteenth century.[16] Chairs of pharmacology were established at the University of Michigan, at Johns Hopkins University and elsewhere.[17] The growth of the Society for Pharmacology and Experimental Therapeutics[18] with academics who joined after the war was significantly spurred on by interest in Salvarsan and chemotherapy.

The career of medical academics was also slowly changing. One of the few really new suggestions of the Flexner Report of 1910 was that medical schools should rely on full-time teaching staff, rather than the lecturers who taught in the schools in addition to their normal practice and other outside activities.[19] By the mid-1920s this suggestion was just beginning to take effect and some of the leading eastern medical schools began to maintain full-time teaching staffs.[20] The trend towards full-time teaching coincided with the movement toward larger and more stable company laboratories. Physicians who had worked both in medical schools and pharmaceutical companies now more often had to choose between them.[21]

The choice was made somewhat easier because companies began to recruit directly. This pattern was most evident at the University of Michigan, fostered by the longstanding ties between the medical school and science departments and Parke Davis.[22] By the post-war period the company was sponsoring a number of students and research projects and expecting many of them eventually to work for the firm.[23] The University of Pennsylvania had a somewhat similar tradition, but the closer ties among the Philadelphia College of Pharmacy, Mulford, and Smith Kline and French formed the most important link in the city between medical schools and the large drug manufacturers.[24]

The new pattern meant that companies could draw upon the large number of science graduates now emerging from college. Their staffs had the potential, therefore, to expand rapidly and they began to be used in the concentration of the industry.

CONCENTRATION

Concentration took two forms in the drug industry. The large producers who in the pre-war years had offered thousands of items became increasingly specialised. Furthermore, there was now a strong incentive for those small firms that wished to continue in the ethical pharmaceuticals business to merge with large companies. There was a significant merger wave in American industry generally during the post-war period and drug makers were very much a part of it. Although business was good and opportunities for expansion existed, many manufacturers lacked the corporate structure to cope with increased size, complicated government regulations and scientific complexity. Many of the firms who made up the American Pharmaceutical Manufacturers' Association in the early 1920s failed to survive the decade.[25]

Most of the major producers drastically cut back the range of products manufactured and carried. Smith Kline and French, for example, reduced their offerings from around 6000 items to 200, discarding much of their patent medicine line and most items which competitors were able to produce at greater profit.[26] Pharmacists were finding it increasingly easy to order their stocks from a few wholesalers or jobbers, and manufacturers sought to avoid problems of mass producing and marketing more than a few items, especially those which required explanation. Sharp and Dohme similarly reduced their range of drugs.[27] Parke Davis and Mulford also cut back their ranges of production,[28] though not as drastically as Smith Kline and French because they had already become quite specialised. Regulations from the Food and Drug Administration made the handling of drugs very different from the early 1890s. Before regulation a firm could base its advertising, as did Parke Davis, only on the fact that a score of their packaged medicines had been standardised.[29]

At Smith Kline and French, Mahlon Kline quickly persuaded the company to focus on the concerns of the laboratory rather than the less profitable business of full-line supplying to pharmacies.[30] The consolidation of the product line disrupted business far less than might be imagined. The most vigorously advertised products, and those with the largest profit margins, now became those enhanced by laboratory science. The best example of this was the Eskay line of baby foods and dietary supplements.[31] Joseph England had devised an early formula for the milk-based baby food, to be given under the directions of a doctor.[32] The move to step up promotion of Eskay products was part of an effort to ally the company more closely with the medical profession.[33] In a widespread battle during the 1920s, baby food makers moved their marketing thrust from a concentration on selling to mothers to using physicians as intermediaries who prescribed and monitored infants' diets. This both expanded the domain of physicians into an area which had previously been the mothers' independent concern, and strengthened the ties these manufacturers held with physicians.[34]

For Smith Kline the success of the Eskay line led the way in a new marketing approach towards physicians. In effect the company had discovered how to make the transition from a wholesaler of patent and proprietary medicines, such as Hand's cures, to ethical pharmaceuticals and to strengthen their reputation as a friend of the profession. The company's reshaped image paralleled its new business structure. While the range of product offerings was being limited, the status of the laboratory was enhanced. Mahlon Kline was better able, after the war, to revise the structure of the laboratory, expanding its staff and encouraging more development work.[35]

The merger movement helped to concentrate the industry further. Among drug makers this was led by the joining of Abbott and DRL in 1922 and culminated in 1929, just before the crash on Wall Street, when the H. K. Mulford Company merged with Sharp and Dohme.[36] The latter marriage joined a leading producer of science-based medicines with a major marketing firm, a leader in wholesale marketing and distribution. The combination of reputation and efficient structure was heralded in the industry as creating the company with the greatest potential to lead the market for the widest range of products.[37] It was a triumph for a pioneer producer and a bold move on the part of Sharp and Dohme.

The merger brought the companies together in a harmonious arrangement. Mulford's managers were appointed to the top board of Sharp and Dohme and most of the middle management remained intact in both companies.[38] Shares in Sharp and Dohme were parcelled out accordingly and the pay of Mulford's directors was increased.[39] Mulford also maintained its corporate identity to a large extent. Its successful products were mostly continued, and all of the Glenolden plant with its biologicals and research staff was left intact.[40] As with Abbott's acquisition of DRL, the main purpose of the combination was to expand the scientific staff of the purchaser.[41] Sharp and Dohme had previously established a basic laboratory only for testing, standardising and quality control of its repackaged and manufactured products.[42] Shortly before the purchase of Mulford assets, the Sharp and Dohme laboratories collaborated with Baltimore scientists in the synthesis of general antiseptics, at the time a lucrative corner of the business, despite being highly competitive.[43] Marketing first within the Baltimore medical community, Sharp and Dohme developed its own antiseptic lozenges and first-aid solutions. Although development results were profitable, they were of a very routine sort and not the stuff of which scientific reputations were made.[44] In fact, the company was just beginning to feel itself fall behind its more technically advanced competitors and to recognise the significance of that backwardness. Mulford at the time of the merger had a scientific staff of over one hundred, with almost a thousand other employees at Glenolden working on the production of biologicals.[45] Although no longer unique among drug makers, Mulford's scientific staff retained its reputation as a leading group.

The chain drugstore movement was one other force which led to consolidation in the drug industry. In the decade 1920–30 the number of drugstores tripled and threatened large wholesalers by their organised buying and, in some cases, manufacturing.[46] The largest combination of this sort at the time was Drugs Incorporated, the result of a merger between Sterling Products Company and the United Drug Company. Sterling continued to manufacture, while United controlled the retail units.[47] This trend finally separated out those companies which were to concentrate on wholesaling and producing proprietary medicines from those which based their businesses on ethical pharmaceuticals.

During the Second World War the drug industry was challenged to produce penicillin on a large scale.[48] The use of antibiotics radically altered therapeutics; it also fundamentally affected the drug manufacturers. The production of antibiotics was ordinarily more complex than that of the biologicals or even chemotherapeutics, and hence even larger and more highly trained scientific staffs had to be assembled.[49]

Moreover, the subsequent search for other antibiotic drugs necessitated creative fundamental research and product development on a greater scale than ever before.[50] Their proliferation was then matched by those of the psychoactive drugs of the 1950s.[51] But none of this was unprecedented. The company structure in which this took place, the laboratories and testing facilities, even the special relationships between marketing departments and physicians had all been established in the years preceding the Great Depression.

Notes

CHAPTER 1

1. The drug industry has attracted only slight attention from business and medical historians. Recent works have included some considerations of limited scope. See Glenn Porter and Harold Livesay, *Merchants and Manufacturers: Studies in the Changing Structure of Nineteenth Century Marketing* (Baltimore: Johns Hopkins University Press, 1971); and Alfred D. Chandler, Jr, *The Visible Hand. The Managerial Revolution in American Business* (Cambridge, Mass.: Harvard University Press, 1977) for a few comments which place the nineteenth century drug merchants into the broadest context of American economic development. Historians of medicine have been even more remiss, though at least one general history gives us some idea of the role of drug makers: see Erwin H. Ackerknecht, *Therapeutics from the Primitives to the Twentieth Century* (New York: Hafner Press, 1973); and Oswei Temkin has some insights in 'Historical Aspects of Drug Therapy', in Paul Talalay (ed.) *Drugs in Our Society* (Baltimore: Johns Hopkins University Press, 1964) pp. 3–16. Any mention of drug manufacturers was probably scorned at the time Fielding H. Garrison wrote *An Introduction to the History of Medicine*, 4th ed., (Philadelphia: W. B. Saunders, 1929); and perhaps this also explains Richard Shryock's single, short paragraph in *The Development of Modern Medicine. An Interpretation of the Social and Scientific Factors Involved* (Madison: University of Wisconsin Press, 1947, reprinted 1979); even though his comments point to the significance of the industry for bacteriology and immunology. Peter Temin's peculiar neglect of the companies in his history of drug regulation is even more surprising, see Peter Temin, *Taking Your Medicine. Drug Regulation in the United States* (Cambridge, Mass.: Harvard University Press, 1980). The imaginative science to come from drug company laboratories is celebrated in such general histories as John Thomas Mahoney, *The Merchants of Life. An Account of the American Pharmaceutical Industry* (New York: Harper, 1959) as well as being heralded in advertising. On the profitability of drug companies, the Fortune 500 listing of major corporations by net profit after taxes usually puts ten or more in the top fifty by percentage of invested capital, or by percentage of sales. Of Philadelphia-based firms alone, the 1958 rankings by invested capital show American Home Products Corporation (which includes Wyeth Laboratories) first, Smith

Kline and French Laboratories second, Warner-Lambert Pharmaceutical Company twenty-ninth. Merck and Company (now based in New Jersey), a firm built on early Philadelphia manufacturers, ranked fiftieth (*Fortune* 500, 1958). See also Walter Measday, 'Pharmaceutical Industry', in Walter Adams (ed.) *The Structure of American Industry* (New York: Macmillan, 1977) pp. 250–84. In the 1980 *Fortune* list (5 May 1980) pp. 274–301 pharmaceutical companies (industrial group 42) had the highest median return on sales (8.9 per cent), led by Smith Kline (17.3 per cent), Merck (16.0 per cent) and Schering Plough (15.5 per cent). Fifteen drug makers were among the top 500 industrials, including American Home Products (99th), Warner-Lambert (105th), Brystol-Myers (122nd), Pfizer (123rd), Merck (147th), Eli Lilly (163rd), Squibb (188th), and Abbott Laboratories (197th). See also David Schwartzman, *Innovation in the Pharmaceutical Industry* (Baltimore: Johns Hopkins University Press, 1976) pp. 76–80.

2. See Robert H. Wiebe, *The Search for Order 1877–1920* (New York: Hill and Wang, 1967) and Glenn Porter, *The Rise of Big Business 1860–1918* (New York: Crowell, 1973). For medicine during the period see James G. Burrow, *Organized Medicine in the Progressive Era. The Move Toward Monopoly* (Baltimore: Johns Hopkins University Press, 1977).

3. Where mentioned in standard histories, a critical view is rarely taken. One exception to this is Ackerknecht, *Therapeutics*, see, for example, pp. 124–5: 'Pharmaceutical industry is as profitable as it is important and useful. Its attempts to present itself to the public as a purely philanthropic or scientific enterprise are sometimes rather annoying.' Even so, Ackerknecht spends no more than two pages on the industry in a book devoted to the history of therapeutics. Shryock, *Development of Modern Medicine*, p. 434, deals with drug companies and scientific research in one paragraph: 'Meanwhile the development of immunology and of experimental pharmacology had promoted the evolution of small drug concerns into large pharmaceutical houses. . . .'

4. See, for example, Seymour E. Horns, *Economics of American Medicine* (New York: Macmillan, 1964).

5. See Wiebe, *Search for Order*; Chandler, *Visible Hand*.

6. Fast-action tableting machines helped to boost the level of mass production of some drugs; chemical and physiological research led to new products. These changes altered the industry fundamentally while large-scale corporate reorganisations have been less profound.

7. The drug companies also relied on semi-skilled workers, usually women, to process and package medicines under sterile conditions. Rows of women were frequently pictured in pamphlets from the companies, mostly working with advanced products. See, for example, 'Mulford in War and Peace', Pamphlet in the Library of Congress; 'A Tour of the Glenolden Plant' in the Mulford Collection, Merck and Company, West Point, Pennsylvania.

8. See, for example, Temin, *Taking Your Medicine*, Chapter 4.

9. Their place within the medical community was a critical factor in the evolution of drug makers into a science-based industry. Philadelphia has been studied as a medical community in a number of historical and

sociological studies. See, for example, James H. S. Bossard, 'A Sociologist Looks at the Doctors', *College of Physicians of Philadelphia, Transactions*, (1937) pp. 1–10, and Leo O'Hara, 'An Emerging Profession, Philadelphia Medicine, 1860–1900', PhD dissertation, University of Pennsylvania, 1976.

10. The leading manufacturers in Philadelphia were: Smith Kline and French, John Wyeth and Sons, and H. K. Mulford. Of secondary importance were Warner Pharmaceutical Company, Shoemaker and Sons, and Powers and Weightman.

11. The case of Parke Davis and its ties with the University of Michigan are discussed later. While some New York manufacturers were well regarded in that city's medical community, they never seem to have formed a coherent group.

12. There were, for example, many similarities in the development of Parke Davis in Detroit and Mulford in Philadelphia.

13. See George Washington Corner, *Two Centuries of Medicine, A History of the School of Medicine, University of Pennsylvania* (Philadelphia, J. B. Lippincott, 1965); and O'Hara, 'Philadelphia Medicine'.

14. Parke Davis, and E. R. Squibb to a slightly lesser extent, have received some scholarly attention. See Peter Steckl, 'Biological Standardization of Drugs before 1928', PhD dissertation, University of Wisconsin, 1969; and Malcolm Weikl, 'Research as a Function of the Pharmaceutical Industry', MA thesis, University of Wisconsin, 1962, both based primarily on Parke Davis material.

15. Public health laboratories which made antitoxin were drug manufacturers. Some, New York in particular, not only produced large quantities of the medicine but also operated as commercial suppliers in competition with other manufacturers.

16. This was, of course, the period when some other industries instituted research and development. In the electrical industry, for example, laboratories were built by General Electric, RCA and Marconi. More pertinently, chemical companies in Germany had, by 1890, built extensive research departments. See Kendall Birr, *Pioneering Industrial Research* (Washington, DC: Public Affairs Press, 1957). Hugh Aiken, *Syntony and Spark. The Origins of Radio* (New York: Wiley, 1976).

17. The best general history of American pharmacy is the Glen Sonnedecker edition of Edward Kremers and George Urdang, *History of Pharmacy*, 4th ed. (Philadelphia: Lippincott, 1976).

18. The term 'ethical pharmaceuticals' came into use after the turn of the century and first seemed to mean 'honest'. Later it was generally defined as medicines not advertised to the public, in contrast to 'patent medicines'. Patent medicines were, of course, rarely patented. They relied on secret formulas to protect their markets. See James Harvey Young, *The Toadstool Millionaires: A Social History of Patent Medicines in America Before Federal Regulation* (Princeton: Princeton University Press, 1961).

19. Industrial research was used in other industries for a similar range of purposes. Some companies, for example, were particularly concerned about patenting around product lines to protect them. See Leonard S. Reich, 'Radio Electronics and the Development of Industrial Research in

the Bell System', PhD dissertation, Johns Hopkins University, 1977.

20. A sense of the physician's demand is clearly evident in Sinclair Lewis, *Martin Arrowsmith* (London: Jonathan Cape, 1925).

21. United States Bureau of the Census, *Twelfth Census (1900), Manufacturers Part I*, Vol. III (Washington, DC: US Census Office, 1902).

22. William Becker, 'Wholesalers of Hardware and Drugs, 1870–1900', PhD dissertation, Johns Hopkins University, 1969, pp. 170–1.

23. In writing a dissertation in economic history, Becker is most concerned with describing the function of wholesalers as economic intermediaries. He concentrates on their marketing functions and growth.

24. George Winston Smith, *Medicines for the Union Army* (Madison: American Institute for the History of Pharmacy, 1962) p. 60; Roscoe C. Clark, *Threescore Years and Ten, A History of Eli Lilly and Company* (Columbia: Lilly, 1964) p. 22.

25. Mulford's first tableting machine (Oberlin Smith and Henry K. Mulford, US Patent No. 413 310, 'Machine for Manufacturing Compressed Pills', 22 October 1889) was crucial in the company's early days for competing with less effectively mechanised producers. See F. E. Stewart, 'Mulford Growth Shows Great Achievement', *Northwestern Druggist* (December 1922) pp. 14–17.

26. Lawrence G. Blochman, *Doctor Squibb* (New York: Simon and Schuster, 1958) pp. 208*ff*. George Winston Smith, (ed.) 'The Squibb Laboratory in 1863', *Journal of the History of Medicine and Allied Sciences*, 13 (1950) pp. 382–94.

27. On the Philadelphia chemical industry see Williams Haynes, *The Chemical Industry* (New York: Van Nostrand, 1954).

28. Mulford, Upjohn, Pfizer and others were still very small manufacturing pharmacies in the 1890s. Lederle Laboratories, formed in 1904, was able to capture one secure market based on antitoxins. See Mahoney, *The Merchants of Life*, p. 163 for Lederle. The actual size of these relatively small companies is difficult to determine since records of assets and number of employees are not always available. Typical of pharmaceutical manufacturers was Charles Pfizer and Company. Formed in 1849, it employed fewer than 200 people after the turn of the century. In 1891 its inventory value was estimated at about \$238 700, and in 1900 it was incorporated with \$100 000 in authorised capital. In 1906 sales amounted to \$3 441 000. Samuel Miles, *Pfizer . . . An Informal History* (New York: Pfizer, 1978) p. 9. The Lilly company was of similar size. It was incorporated in 1881 and capitalised at \$40 000 and in 1899 sales came to \$423 000. E. J. Kahn, *All in a Century, The First 100 Years of Eli Lilly and Company* (Indianapolis: Eli Lilly, 1976) pp. 23, 35. Upjohn started in 1887 with capital stock of \$60 000 but failed to expand as quickly as its competitors. Haynes, *Chemical Industry*, vol. 3, p. 455. Parke Davis was incorporated in 1875 with capital of \$81 950 and grew to be one of the world's largest pharmaceutical manufacturers by the end of the century. Sales averaged \$3.2 million a year between 1892 and 1901. Haynes, ibid., p. 320 and Mahoney, *Merchants of Life*, pp. 72–3. In Philadelphia only Smith Kline and French was anywhere near that size. Formed by a series of mergers, the last in 1891, the company reached \$3 million in sales in

1902. Tobias Wagner, 'A Story of Growth', unpublished manuscript, c. 1966, SmithKline Archives.

29. Experimentation on new combinations accounted for most of the research effort at Parke Davis and Smith Kline and French. This is readily apparent in *Scientific Contributions from the Laboratories 1866–1966* (Detroit: Parke Davis, 1966) and *Report of the Analytical Laboratory, Smith Kline and French* (Philadelphia: Smith Kline and French, 1904) in SmithKline Archives.

30. Figures on total investment in scientific work are not available but drug companies were forced to establish laboratories after the regulatory acts of 1902 and 1906, after which they became increasingly important for competition with other firms.

31. On the history of pharmacopoeiae, see Kremers and Urdang, *History of Pharmacy*, pp. 260–8.

32. Chandler, *Visible Hand*, pp. 219–21.

33. Becker, 'Wholesalers', p. 170.

34. Ibid., p. 171.

35. Mulford and Parke Davis were masters of image-building.

36. Formal, organised science in the second half of the nineteenth century was growing into a professional, laboratory-based pursuit. It was this image of science which was presented by companies when they wished to show their enlightenment.

37. See, for example, John J. Beer, 'Coal Tar Dye Manufacture and the Origins of the Modern Industrial Research Laboratory', *Isis*, 49 (1958) pp. 123–31.

38. Early scientific activity at Parke Davis, for example, was collecting and classifying; see Chapter 2. This tradition had fallen away for the most part by 1895 when laboratories were built, although the H. K. Mulford Company sponsored a botanical expedition in the style of the previous century in 1921–2, when they backed Henry H. Rusby, a Columbia University botanist, on an Amazon expedition. See file 'Rusby, H. H., M.D., Description of New Genera and Species of Plants Collected on the Mulford Biological Exploration of the Amazon Valley, 1921–1922', Mulford papers. See also George A. Bender, 'Henry Hurd Rusby', *Pharmacy in History*, 23 (1981) pp. 71–85.

39. Robert H. Wiebe, *The Search for Order 1877–1920* (New York: Hill and Wang, 1967) pp. 113–16.

40. See, for example, Rene Vallery-Radot, *The Life of Pasteur* (New York: Sun Dial Press, 1937) Chap. XII, pp. 390*ff*.

41. Mahoney, *Merchants of Life*, pp. 1–4; Temin, *Taking Your Medicine*, p. 58.

42. Richard H. Shryock, *The Development of Modern Medicine, An Interpretation of the Social and Scientific Factors Involved* (Madison: University of Wisconsin Press, 1974) pp. 294*ff*.

43. See, for example, Anon., *How to Succeed as a Physician, Heart to Heart Talks of a Successful Physician with his Brother Practitioners* (Meriden, Conn: Church Pub. Co., 1902) pp. 94–96.

44. Selman Waksman, who later gained fame for his work on antibiotics, worked in a company producing serums before the First World War and

gained greatly from the experience. 'The two years that I spent at the commercial company [Cutter Laboratories] suggested to me new ideas, new approaches, and especially new tools for further study and for broadening the whole field of microbiology.' Waksman spent the rest of his life on producing new drugs both inside and outside companies. Selman A. Waksman, *My Life with the Microbes* (London: Scientific Book Club, 1958) pp. 89–90, 95–8, 295.

45. The US Hygienic Laboratory required a 'responsible head' for vaccine producers. This person had to be trained in bacteriology and either medicine or veterinary science. See National Archives, Record Group 90, Public Health Service Hygienic Laboratory, General File 3655, Box 340–341, on the administration of early government regulations.

46. Mulford used their staff to maintain close contact with the Philadelphia College of Pharmacy. See 'A Visit to the H. K. Mulford Company', *Philadelphia College of Pharmacy, Alumni Report*, 35 (1899) pp. 252–57; A. Fabian and W. H. Guest, 'A Vist to the Bacteriologic Laboratories of the H. K. Mulford Company', *Alumni Report*, 36 (1900) pp. 30–4.

47. The term 'high technology' may seem somewhat anachronistic but corresponds well to the self-image of drug companies. A comparison of Mulford's or the Dermatological Research Laboratory's promotional material with that of, say, Bell Laboratories shows this similarity.

48. This contrast was all the more apparent in its absence, since patent medicine makers were rarely acknowledged in company materials. The lobbying for standardisation was clearly directed against patent medicine competitors.

49. Mulford marketed a meningitis serum in 1901. See Mulford Bulletin No. 8, 'Antimeningitis Serum' (Philadelphia: Mulford, n.d.). In 1926 confirmation of the inefficiency of the serum was published.

50. Very few American drug producers used patents for their medicines, although they routinely patented mechanical devices such as syringes, drug cases and vaccine shields.

51. On the development of a strategy of patent use by German chemical companies, see J. Liebenau, 'Patents in the Chemical Industry', in *The Challenge of New Technology* (London: Gower, 1987).

52. See Reich, 'Radio Electronics', on electrical manufacturers. On the general use of patents at the turn of the century see Story B. Ladd, 'Patents in Relation to Manufacturers', *United States Census 1900*, Vol. 10, Manufacturers, No. 4, Selected Industries (Washington DC: USPGO, 1902).

53. The Hoechst company lawyers supplied their scientists with standard forms to fill out to apply for an American patent. These would then be processed by a New York patent attorney.

54. Behring's patent application: No. 606 042, National Archives, Patent Records.

55. Mulford and Parke Davis employed something of the order of 30 trained scientists at any one time by the end of the century.

56. Steckl, 'Biological Standardization'.

57. Mulford offered a prize for outstanding students at the Philadelphia College of Pharmacy. See Joseph England (ed.) *The First Century of the*

Philadelphia College of Pharmacy, 1821–1921 (Philadelphia: Philadelphia College of Pharmacy, 1922). They also allowed the students to take frequent tours around their plant (*Philadelphia College of Pharmacy, Alumni Reports,* of 1896, 1897, 1899, etc.) and maintained a herb garden for the school. See 'Correspondence, Philadelphia College of Pharmacy and Mulford – Glenolden site', 1925, file in Mulford papers.

58. All the associates of the Dermatological Research Laboratory were in the faculty of the University of Pennsylvania Medical School and continued to teach while working at the company. Herman Metz supplied funds for research at Columbia by Levy, Hooper and Funk.

59. Most physicians working in the companies maintained their affiliations at local hospitals. Philadelphia firms relied on their contacts at the Pennsylvania Hospital, the Philadelphia General Hospital and the German (now Lankenau) Hospital.

60. See, for example, Mulford, 'Price List', 1900, in Smithsonian Institution, pp. 535, 545, where University (of Pennsylvania) Hospital and Roosevelt Hospital (New York) are named.

61. Experts were often lured away with higher wages, more research freedom or opportunities to study for further degrees or to gain medical training. This was the case with Pearson and Kebler at Smith Kline, who both earned MDs while working for the company, and were lured by this prospect, respectively, away from H. M. Alexander's and Parke Davis.

62. The inadequacy of the literature for explaining actual chemical processes was much commented upon. When the Dermatological Research Laboratory tried to produce Salvarsan they were frustrated by the inadequacy of the patent and the literature on its production.

63. Salaries were usually above the standard $2000–$3000 per year these men might earn in public health laboratories. See *Philadelphia Board of Health, Annual Report* (1894), p. 127 for Joseph McFarland's salary as head of the bacteriological laboratory. He earned at least another $2000 by joining Mulford. McFarland papers Box II, College of Physicians of Philadelphia.

64. Lewis, *Martin Arrowsmith*, p. 148.

65. Ibid., pp. 150–1.

66. Ibid., p. 150.

67. Ibid., pp. 292*ff*, 315*ff*, 345*ff*.

68. This is developed in J. Liebenau, 'Medicine and Technology', *Perspectives in Biology and Medicine*, 27 (1983).

CHAPTER 2

1. In this short period of growth after the economic disruption of the war of 1812–15, coupled with the decline in British commerce as a result of the Napoleonic Wars, a large number of manufacturing firms were established, including the predecessors of some of the major chemical manufacturers of the end of the century. Three companies later to form the Philadelphia base of Sharp and Dohme (subsequently Merck and

Company) date from this period: Farr and Kunzi (1818), Powers and Weightman (1818) and Rosengarten and Sons (1821/22). The Marshall Drug Store, which had been established at the end of the previous century, grew into a manufacturing house at this time and led a wave of conversions from retail pharmacies to wholesale and manufacturing businesses, and Charles V. Hagner operated a 'drug mill' starting in 1812, but it was not until 1817 that he began producing his more significant products, verdigris and white lead, for which he received process patents in that year. John and Daniel Elliott began their fine chemical manufacturing in 1819. See: J. Thomas Scharf and Thompson Westcott, *History of Philadelphia 1609–1884* (Philadelphia: L. H. Evans, 1884) p. 2234; John J. MacFarlane, *Manufacturing in Philadelphia 1683–1912* (Philadelphia: Philadelphia Commercial Museum, 1912) pp. 63–4. See also Edward Kremers and George Urdang, *History of Pharmacy*, 4th ed. (Philadephia: Lippincott, 1976) pp. 181–212, 226–31, 326–35; and John Thomas Mahoney, *The Merchants of Life. An Account of the American Pharmaceutical Industry* (New York: Harper, 1959) pp. 30–1. The best general source on pharmacy in Philadelphia is Joseph W. England (ed.) *The First Century of the Philadelphia College of Pharmacy 1821–1921* (Philadelphia: Philadelphia College of Pharmacy, 1922).

2. This was so even in the context of a major agricultural depression and general paralysis of industry. In this early period, drug manufacturing responded economically more to import levels than to other factors. For the extent of the decline, which reached its nadir in 1819, see Scharf and Westcott, *History of Philadelphia*, p. 2234.

3. Drugs were powdered by hand in large mortars and pills were rolled out and dried previous to sale. Tinctures were made by maceration (soaking) and expression (squeezing) and crude drugs were treated with chemicals, often alcohol, to extract soluble products. Bandages were made by applying a coating to rough cloth. See, for example, Kremers and Urdang, *History of Pharmacy*, pp. 181*ff*. Also England, *Philadelphia College of Pharmacy*, pp. 114–15, on percolation.

4. In aggregate, the profits of drug makers have been high during the entire period over which the US census has counted income. United States Bureau of the Census, *Ninth Census of Manufacturers* (Washington: US Census Office, 1880).

5. 'Report from America', *Medical Times and Gazette* (London) 1872i, p. 109.

6. England, *Philadelphia College of Pharmacy*, pp. 36, 136, 355–6. Kremers and Urdang, *History of Pharmacy*, pp. 326–7.

7. Williams Haynes, *American Chemical Industry*, vol. 1 (New York: Van Nostrand, 1954) p. 211.

8. Mahoney, *Merchants of Life*, p. 8.

9. Ibid., pp. 30–1.

10. England, *Philadelphia College of Pharmacy*, p. 33.

11. Ibid., p. 111. Artifacts from almost one hundred years of the production of Seidlitz powders in the United States can be seen in the Division of Medical Sciences, National Museum of American History, Smithsonian

Institution, Washington, DC.

12. England, *Philadelphia College of Pharmacy*, pp. 31–35.
13. Ibid., pp. 110–12.
14. For example, Erwin H. Ackerknecht, *Therapeutics from the Primitives to the Twentieth Century* (New York: Hafner, 1973) p. 99, identifies a constant close connection between drugs and either rational theory or empiricism in the early nineteenth century, but one only has to look at the popular patent medicines to see that the connection with either theory or experience was often highly tenuous. See James Harvey Young, *American Self-Dosage Medicines. An Historical Perspective* (Lawrence, Kansas: Coronado Press, 1974) pp. 1–13; also J. H. Young, *The Toadstool Millionaires. A Social History of Patent Medicines in America Before Federal Regulation* (Princeton: Princeton University Press, 1961).
15. Charles E. Rosenberg, 'The Therapeutic Revolution: Medicine, Meaning and Social Change in Nineteenth-Century America', in Morris J. Vogel and Charles E. Rosenberg (eds) *The Therapeutic Revolution, Essays in the Social History of American Medicine* (Philadelphia: University of Pennsylvania Press, 1979) pp. 7–9.
16. See George Rosen, *Fees and Fee Bills* (Baltimore: Johns Hopkins University Press, 1946) pp. 1–3. Also William G. Rothstein, *American Physicians in the Nineteenth Century, From Sects to Science* (Baltimore: Johns Hopkins University Press, 1972) pp. 63–4.
17. Foremost, see Rosenberg, 'Therapeutic Revolution.' See also Gert Brieger, 'Therapeutic Conflict and the American Medical Profession in the 1860s', *Bulletin of the History of Medicine*, 41 (1967) pp. 215–23. For a general history of the shift from heroic therapeutics, see Ackerknecht, *Therapeutics*, pp. 118–19. Also Alex Berman, 'The Heroic Approach in 19th Century Therapeutics', *Bulletin of the American Society of Hospital Pharmacists* (1954) pp. 320–7; Guenter B. Risse, 'The Brownian System of Medicine: Its Theoretical and Practical Implications', *Clio Medica*, 5 (1970) pp. 45–51; Harris L. Coulter, *Divided Legacy: A History of the Schism in Medical Thought*, 3 vols, (Washington, DC: American Institute of Homeopathy, 1973); Rothstein, *American Physicians*, pp. 41–55, 152–74, 230–246; Joseph F. Kett, *The Formation of the American Medical Profession. The Role of Institutions, 1780–1860* (New Haven: Yale University Press, 1968) pp. 132–64; John S. Haller, 'The Use and Abuse of Tartar Emetic in the 19th Century Materia Medica', *Bulletin of the History of Medicine*, 49 (1975) pp. 235–57; Guenter B. Risse, 'The Renaissance of Bloodletting: A Chapter in Modern Therapeutics', *Journal of the History of Medicine and Allied Sciences*, 34 (1979) pp. 3–22; John Harley Warner, '"The Nature-Trusting Heresy": American Physicians and the Concept of the Healing Power of Nature in the 1850s and 1860s', *Perspectives in American History*, 11 (1977–78) pp. 298–324; and John Harley Warner, 'Physiological Theory and Therapeutic Explanation in the 1860s: The British Debate on the Medical Use of Alcohol', *Bulletin of the History of Medicine*, 54 (1980) pp. 235–57; and 'Therapeutic Explanation and the Edinburgh Blood-letting Controversy: Two Perspectives on the Medical Meaning of

Science in the Mid-Nineteenth Century', *Medical History* (1980) pp. 241–58.

18. Rosenberg, 'Therapeutic Revolution', p. 6.

19. The range of their effects can be seen in the organisation of materia medica texts: they were usually not arranged according to drug or disease, but as diuretics, cathartics, narcotics, emetics, etc. – that is, by drug action.

20. 'Report from America', *Medical Times and Gazette*. See also Rosenberg, 'Therapeutic Revolution', p. 13.

21. Young, *Toadstool Millionaires*, p. 78; Rosenberg, 'Therapeutic Revolution', p. 9; and Brieger, 'Therapeutic Conflict', pp. 215–22.

22. Rothstein, *American Physicians*, p. 139; Young, *Self-Dosage Medicines*, p. 4; and 'Patent Medicines and the Self-Help Syndrome', in Guenter B. Risse, Ronald L. Numbers, and Judith Walzer Leavitt, *Medicine Without Doctors, Home Health Care in American History* (New York: Science History Publications, 1977) pp. 95–116.

23. This was particularly true, for example, at Smith Kline and at Wyeth.

24. 'Report on the Drug Trade', *Proceedings of the Annual Convention of the American Pharmaceutical Association, 1879*, pp. 551–61.

25. T. Salmon, 'Prescribing by Druggists, and the Remedy,' *Medical Register* (Philadelphia) 1887i, p. 323.

26. Kremers and Urdang, *History of Pharmacy*, p. 180. J. R. Lothrop, 'Verdict Against an Apothecary for an Alleged Mistake in Putting up a Prescription', *Buffalo Medical and Surgical Journal*, 6 (1886–7) pp. 85, 117, 343; 'Important Action by the Philadelphia County Medical Society in Relation to Certain Objectionable Practices by Druggists, Injurious to the Interests of Medical Practitioners', *College and Clinical Record* (Philadelphia) 1881i, p. 19.

27. Kremers and Urdang, *History of Pharmacy*, p. 180.

28. 'Report from America', *Medical Times and Gazette*.

29. Ibid.

30. Scharf and Westcott, *History of Philadelphia*, p. 2249. See also James Harvey Young, 'Pioneer Nostrum Promoter: Thomas W. Dyott', *Journal of the American Pharmaceutical Association*, n.s. 1 (1961) p. 290.

31. A flamboyant person, Dyott established a Christian Utopia called Dyottville out of his drug mill and glass works in which 300 persons worked. Over 200 of these were 'apprentices' whose lives he ruled through strict moral guidelines. One aspect of this policy ironically helped lead to his failure during the depression of 1837: 'In order to encourage saving habits, he established a bank at his former drug-store, Second and Race Streets, which was called the Manual Labor Bank. . . . He succeeded in obtaining large deposits on promise to pay interest, pushed his notes into extensive circulation, and, when the day of distrust came, and he was called upon to redeem his notes, he could not respond.' Scharf and Westcott, *History of Philadelphia*, p. 2249.

32. Young, *Toadstool Millionaires*, p. 112; quoted from Dr Euen, *An Essay in the Form of a Lecture, on Political and Medical Quackery* (Philadelphia: c. 1845).

33. Young, *Toadstool Millionaires*, pp. 35, 75–85.

34. Scharf and Westcott, *History of Philadelphia*, p. 2249. Young, *Toadstool Millionaires*, pp. 35–6.
35. England, *Philadelphia College of Pharmacy*, p. 107.
36. Ibid., p. 108.
37. John F. Marion, *The Fine Old House. The History of SmithKline Corp.* (Philadelphia: SmithKline, 1980).
38. Ibid.
39. Ibid.
40. Philadelphia City Directory, 1841.
41. Marion, *SmithKline*.
42. Young, *Toadstool Millionaires*; William Becker, 'Wholesalers of Hardware and Drugs, 1870–1900', PhD dissertation, Johns Hopkins University, 1969.
43. Ibid.; see also Glenn Porter and Harold Livesay, *Merchants and Manufacturers: Studies in the Changing Structure of Nineteenth Century Marketing* (Baltimore: Johns Hopkins University Press, 1974) p. 29.
44. Ibid., pp. 29–34. The Troth papers are at the Elutherian Mills, Hagley Foundation Library.
45. Porter and Livesay, *Merchants and Manufacturers*.
46. Ibid., p. 33. Typically of drug merchants, Troth relied on imported, particularly British, goods. Porter and Livesay noted that: 'The Troths bought drugs from import houses such as W. H. Schieffelin and Company, Clark and McConnin, and Cummins and Reach (all of New York), from Baltimore's Smith and Atkinson and Brickhead and Pierce, and from local Philadelphia merchants such as Ziegler and Smith.' Ibid., p. 30.
47. Ibid., p. 34. Samuel Troth to Prichard and Son, 26 July 1843.
48. Ibid., Samuel Troth to Dr N. Marmion, 30 August 1843.
49. Tobias Wagner, 'Smith Kline and French', unpublished, public relations history c. 1961, SmithKline Records, p. 20.
50. Ibid.
51. George Winston Smith (ed.) 'The Squibb Laboratory in 1863', *Journal of the History of Medicine and Allied Sciences*, 13 (1958) pp. 382–94; Lawrence G. Blochman, *Doctor Squibb, The Life and Times of a Rugged Individualist* (New York: Simon and Schuster, 1958) pp. 133–37.
52. George Winston Smith, *Medicines for the Union Army* (Madison: American Institute for the History of Pharmacy, 1962) p. 81; from *A Statement of the Causes Which Led to the Dismissal of Surgeon General William Alexander Hammond from the Army* (New York: n.p., 1864) p. 63. Other major orders went to the Louisville firm Wilson and Peter ($592 809.37) and the New York companies Philip Schieffelin and Company ($306 694.67) and to Squibb ($286 199.40).
53. Smith, *Union Army*, p. 14.
54. 'Report of a Committee of the Boston Society for Medical Improvement, on the Alleged Dangers Which Accompany the Inhalation of the Vapor of Sulphuric Ether', *Boston Medical and Surgical Journal*, 65 (1861) p. 230. See also Smith, 'Squibb, 1863'.
55. Smith, *Union Army*, op. cit., p. 60.
56. Dr Bill's report is perhaps the most detailed description of the structure

and operation of a drug laboratory during the Civil War.

57. Smith, 'Squibb, 1863'.
58. Smith, *Union Army*, p. 60.
59. George D. Rosengarten had an income of $98 526 in 1864, and William D. Weightman earned $83 255; E. Digby Baltzell, *Philadelphia Gentlemen, The Making of a National Upper Class* (Glencoe, Ill.: Free Press, 1958).
60. Chronology, SmithKline Records.
61. United States Bureau of the Census, *Historical Statistics of the United States, Colonial Times to 1970*, part 1 (Washington, DC: USGPO, 1975) p. 210.
62. At the Smithsonian Institution, one can see the effect of this expansion of the function of pharmacies. Artifacts from after the Civil War cover a wide range of items, from brushes and mirrors to candy and cleaning aids.
63. United States Bureau of the Census, *Ninth Census of Manufacturers*, vol. 3 (Washington, DC: US Bureau of the Census, 1870) pp. 394–402.
64. See US Census *Historical Statistics* (1975) p. 210.
65. Ibid.
66. Warner, 'Alcohol'.
67. Brieger, 'Therapeutic Conflict'.
68. The military pharmacy service was well organised during the Civil War. See Smith, *Union Army*, op. cit.; and Kremers and Urdang, *History of Pharmacy*, p. 346. Both the nature of pharmaceutical products (potency, concentration) and the methods of administration (dosage) were affected by these changes.
69. Kremers and Urdang, *History of Pharmacy*, pp. 265–7.
70. Glenn Sonnedecker, 'The Pharmacopoeia and America – 150 Years of Service', *Pharmacy in History*, 12 (1970) pp. 156–9. See also Erika Hickel, *Arzneimittel-Standisierung im 19. Jahrhundert in den Pharmacopoen Deutschlands, Frankreiches, Grossbrittanniens, und der Vereinigten Staaten von Amerika* (Stuttgart: Wissenschaftliche Verlagsgesellschaft, 1973).
71. Ibid.
72. Kremers and Urdang, *History of Pharmacy*, pp. 263–4.
73. Ibid., pp. 263–7.
74. Philadelphia Drug Exchange, Circular No. 49, 10 November 1877 (Historical Society of Pennsylvania).
75. Editorial, *New Remedies* June 1878, p. 162. See also Becker, 'Wholesalers,' p. 173.
76. Kremers and Urdang, *History of Pharmacy*, p. 327.
77. England, *Philadelphia College*, pp. 43–59.
78. *American Journal of Pharmacy*; Kremers and Urdang, *History of Pharmacy*, p. 288.
79. Becker, 'Wholesalers' p. 174.
80. Kremers and Urdang, *History of Pharmacy*, p. 383.
81. Ibid., p. 235. Ten new schools were established in each of the post Civil War decades, twenty in the 1880s and thirty in the 1890s.
82. England, *Philadelphia College*, pp. 130ff, 151–2.

83. Ibid., p. 132.
84. Ibid., pp. 149*ff.* See also 'Licensing of Pharmacists', *Philadelphia Board of Health, Annual Reports, 1880–1920.*
85. Ibid. See also Kremers and Urdang, *History of Pharmacy*, pp. 189–98.
86. Smith, *Union Army*, p. 60.
87. Becker, 'Wholesalers', pp. 185–6.
88. Philadelphia Drug Exchange, Circular No. 49, 10 November 1877 (Historical Society of Pennsylvania, Philadelphia).
89. Ibid.
90. Becker, 'Wholesalers', pp. 185–6.
91. Ibid., p. 187.
92. Fliers in Historical Society of Pennsylvania.
93. Ibid.
94. England, *Philadelphia College*, pp. 32–3; Marion, *SmithKline*.
95. Philadelphia, *Census of Manufacturers of Philadelphia 1882*. See also Scharf and Westcott, *History of Philadelphia*, p. 2246.
96. United States Bureau of the Census, *Tenth Census of Manufacturers, 1880* (Washington, DC: US Bureau of the Census, 1882).
97. Philadelphia, *Census of 1882*.
98. Advertisements and catalogues, SmithKline Records; 'Smith Kline and French', *Pharmaceutical Era* (1893); also Warshaw Collection, Smithsonian Institution.
99. Paul C. Olsen, *The Merchandising of Drug Products* (New York: Appleton, 1931).
100. Alfred D. Chandler, *The Visible Hand. The Managerial Revolution in American Business* (Cambridge, Mass.: Harvard University Press, 1977) pp. 214–15.
101. Ibid.
102. Ibid.
103. 'Smith Kline', *Pharmaceutical Era*; Porter and Livesay, *Merchants and Manufacturers*.
104. 'Smith Kline', *Pharmaceutical Era*.
105. Chandler, *Visible Hand*, pp. 218–19.
106. Collections of pamphlets, Smithsonian Institution.
107. Ibid.
108. George B. Swayze, 'The Professional Relations Between the Physician and the Druggist', *Medical Times* (Philadelphia).
109. C. R. Rorem and R. P. Fischelis, *The Costs of Medicine* (Chicago: Committee on the Costs of Medical Care, 1932).
110. Philadelphia Medical Society, 'Rules, 1877', Library of Congress.
111. Horatio C. Wood, 'Reminiscences of an American Pioneer in Experimental Medicine', *College of Physicians of Philadelphia, Transactions*, 3rd series, 42 (1920) pp. 195–234. See also G. E. de Schweinitz, 'Dr H. C. Wood as a Medical Teacher,' *College of Physicians of Philadelphia Transactions* 3rd series, 42 (1920) pp. 235–241.
112. J. McKeen Cattell and J. Cattell, *American Men of Science*, 5th ed. (New York: The Science Press, 1935) p. 1231.
113. Horatio C. Wood, *A Treatise on Therapeutics, Comprising Materia Medica and Toxicology, with Special Reference to the Application of the*

Physiological Action of Drugs to Clinical Medicine (Philadelphia: Lippincott, 1874). Subsequent editions were printed in 1875, 1879, 1882, 1883, 1885, 1888. The title was then changed to *Therapeutics: Its Principles and Practice: A Word on Medical Agencies, Drugs and Poisons, with Especial Reference to the Relations between Physiology and Clinical Medicine*, which was issued in five editions from 1891–1905.

114. Wood, 'Reminiscences', p. 215.
115. Kremers and Urdang, *History of Pharmacy*.
116. Williams Haynes, *American Chemical Industry*, vol. VI (New York: Van Nostrand, 1954) pp. 271–5; Mahoney, *Merchants of Life*, pp. 191–203. See acquisitions chart in Merck and Company archives, West Point, Pennsylvania.
117. Wood, 'Reminiscences'.
118. J. A. Roth, 'Wood', in *Health Purifiers and Their Enemies* (New York: Neil Watson, 1977).
119. Wood. 'Reminiscences'; Roth, 'Wood'; 'Dr. Wood's Biographical Record'. *College of Physicians of Philadelphia, Transactions*, 3rd series, 42 (1920) pp. 242–57.
120. James Harvey Young, *The Medical Messiahs: A Social History of Health Quackery in Twentieth-Century America* (Princeton: Princeton University Press, 1967) p. 83.
121. See Chapter 9.
122. H. C. Wood, Joseph R. Remington, and Samuel P. Sadler, *The Dispensatory of the United States of America. Rearranged, Thoroughly Revised and Rewritten*, 15th ed. (Philadelphia: Lippincott, 1883).
123. George B. Swayze, *Medical Times* (Philadelphia). Quoted in Leo J. O'Hara, 'Emerging Profession, Philadelphia Medicine, 1860–1900', PhD dissertation, University of Pennsylvania, 1976.
124. United States Census, *Census of 1900*, Vol. 10, Manufacturers, No. 4, Selected Industries (Washington, DC: Census Office, 1902) pp. 612–15.
125. Aimar Pharmacy Records, Smithsonian Institution, Washington, DC.

CHAPTER 3

1. Parke, Davis and Company, *Parke-Davis at 100, Progress in the Past, Promise for the Future, 1866–1966, 100th Aniversay* (Detroit: Parke Davis, 1966); E. J. Kahn, Jr, *All in a Century . . . the First 100 years of Eli Lilly and Co.* (Indianapolis: Eli Lilly and Company, 1976); for Upjohn see: Leonard Engel, *Medicine Makers of Kalamazoo* (New York: Upjohn Corporation, 1961); 'The Upjohn Company' in Williams Haynes, *American Chemical Industry*, Vol. VI (New York: Van Nostrand, 1954) pp. 455–7. Catalogues from these companies are at the Smithsonian Institution.
2. John F. Marion, *The Fine Old House, The History of SmithKline Corporation* (Philadelphia: SmithKline, 1980); 'Smith Kline and French Company', *The Pharmaceutical Era*, 31 December 1896, pp. 995–7.
3. Alfred D. Chandler, Jr, *The Visible Hand. The Managerial Revolution in*

American Business (Cambridge, Mass.: Harvard University Press, 1977).

4. See Glenn Porter, *The Rise of Big Business 1860–1910* (New York: Crowell, 1973) pp. 71–84.
5. United States Bureau of the Census, *Twelfth Census, Census of Manufacturers*, Vol. VII (Washington DC: U.S. Census Office, 1902) pp. 6, 170, 180, 530.
6. Frank O. Taylor, 'Forty-Five Years of Manufacturing Pharmacy', *Journal of the American Pharmaceutical Association*, 4 (1915) pp. 468–81. See also Wyeth advertisements in Wyeth Records, and Smith Kline advertisements in SmithKline Records. See also Tobias Wagner, unpublished history of Smith Kline, in SmithKline Records; 'Smith Kline', *Pharmaceutical Era*; and 'Smith, Kline and French Company Celebrates Its 82nd Birthday', *The North American*, 25 February 1923.
7. Porter, *Big Business*, p. 18.
8. Eli Lilly had an early branch operation when it opened a St Louis plant around 1882. See Kahn, *Eli Lilly*.
9. Efficient warehousing meant a hierarchy of clerks and a smoothly operating packaging and shipping department. Smith Kline was most successful at this, see 'Smith Kline', *Pharmaceutical Era*.
10. Chandler, *Visible Hand*; Porter, *Big Business*, pp. 71*ff*.
11. Marion, *SmithKline*; Haynes, *Chemical Industry*, Vol. VI. Parke Davis and Company had long claimed to be 'the physician's drug supplier', offering 'the highest quality and the best standardized drugs'. It was certainly one of the largest suppliers and manufacturers of high quality drugs by the mid-1890s and dominated trade in the mid-west and west from its plants in and around Detroit. The firm had its origins in mid-century in a sequence of partnerships between physicians and merchants, incorporating in 1875. Through the 1880s Parke Davis concentrated on developing new markets by introducing unique products. As demand grew they expanded their lakeside location and their use of shipping and railways. They also began to specialise in rural sales and assembled extensive catalogues to improve their procedures for soliciting orders. Taylor, 'Forty-Five Years'; Malcolm Keith Weikel, 'Research as a Function of the Pharmaceutical Industry, The American Formative Period', MA thesis, University of Wisconsin, 1962.
12. Most notably Smith Kline, which operated a massive stockroom and shipping department.
13. In particular Mulford, which was organised to promote quick growth.
14. 'Smith Kline', *Pharmaceutical Era*.
15. Parke Davis advertisements and trade catalogues, Smithsonian Institution and the College of Physicians of Philadelphia.
16. Wyeth advertisements, Box D45, Warshaw Collection, Smithsonian Institution.
17. 'Smith Kline', *Pharmaceutical Era*; also claimed in advertisements, Box D45, Warshaw Collection.
18. Photograph, c. 1895, SmithKline Records.
19. Tobias Wagner, 'Smith Kline and French', unpublished public relations history, SmithKline Records.

20. Order books, Aimar Pharmacy Records; Smithsonian Institution, and Receipt Book, SmithKline Records.

21. Joseph W. England (ed.) *The First Century of the Philadelphia College of Pharmacy 1821–1921* (Philadelphia: Philadelphia College of Pharmacy, 1922); Francis E. Stewart, (Mulford Company History) 'Twenty Years, 1891–1911', (H. K. Mulford Papers, Merck and Company Archives, West Point, Pennsylvania). See also Francis E. Stewart, 'Mulford Growth Shows Great Achievment', *Northwestern Druggist*, 30 (1922) pp. 14–17. Henry Mulford received his pharmacy diploma in 1887.

22. C. F. Hayward, 'Growth of the Manufacturing Departments of the H. K. Mulford Company', *Keystone*, 1 (1919) pp. 3–4. The *Keystone* was the Mulford Company newsletter.

23. Stewart, 'Twenty Years'.

24. Stewart, 'Mulford Growth'.

25. *Keystone*, 2 (1919) p. 1.

26. H. M. Alexander's Vaccine Company, papers in the possession of Dr John H. Brown, Marietta, Pennsylvania, hereafter referred to as Alexander Records. Dr John H. Brown, interview, 5 September 1980. Advertisements from the Alexander Company are in the Joseph McFarland Papers, Library of the College of Physicians of Philadelphia (hereafter McFarland Papers) and at the Smithsonian Institution.

27. James Harvey Young, *The Medical Messiahs: A Social History of Health Quackery in Twentieth-Century America* (Princeton: Princeton University Press, 1967) p. 23.

28. US Hygienic Laboratory Records, 1898–1910, National Archives. Collection of reports from inspectors showed the precarious finances of some of the small companies. See also advertisements and catalogues from Pocono Laboratories, Lancaster Vaccine Farm, Slee's Vaccine Farm, and the National Vaccine Establishment, McFarland Papers.

29. Oral History, 13 March 1953, Tom Fehnenberger file, SmithKline Records: 'When Sharp and Dohme moved to Philadelphia their production had a very bad effect on the Philadelphia market and disrupted the operation of many local drug firms. Smith Kline and French Company was forced to take drastic action, and it was announced that all recently employed people would be laid off but older employees would be kept on on a full-time basis.' The employees chose, in this case, to fight to keep the entire workforce and negotiated for a temporary two-day week until the company could return to full production.

30. Sharp and Dohme catalogues in Smithsonian Institution; Smith Kline catalogues in SmithKline Records; Aimar Pharmacy records show extensive ordering from both these suppliers.

31. Collections of catalogues at the College of Physicians of Philadelphia and Smithsonian Institution.

32. Parke Davis based its reputation on its close ties to the medical profession, see Peter Steckl, 'Biological Standardization of Drugs Before 1928', PhD dissertation, University of Wisconsin, 1969. Smith Kline based theirs on their superior distribution system, see 'Smith Kline', *Pharmaceutical Era*; Sterns, Merck and Schieffelin on their imports from Europe; see Merck and Company, 'From Angel Apothecary to World

Wide Nework', (New York: Merck and Company, 1976); see also Chandler, *Visible Hand*, pp. 218–19.

33. Glen Porter, *Big Business*, pp. 71–84; and Ralph L. Nelson, *Merger Movements in American Industry, 1895–1956* (Princeton: Princeton University Press, 1959).

34. See Reese V. Jenkins, *Images and Enterprise: Technology and the American Photographic Industry 1839–1925*, (Baltimore: Johns Hopkins University Press, 1975); and Maurice Corina, *Trust in Tobacco* (London: Joseph, 1975).

35. Peter Temin, *Taking Your Medicine. Drug Regulation in the United States* (Cambridge, Mass.: Harvard University Press, 1980) p. 87.

36. Germany allowed drug-making processes to be patented but France permitted no patents on medicines. Medicines were rarely patented in Great Britain.

37. Young, *The Medical Messiahs*, p. 14.

38. Leonard Reich, 'Radio Electronics and the Development of Industrial Research in the Bell System', PhD dissertation, Johns Hopkins University, 1977, pp. 171–4.

39. US Bureau of the Census, *Twelfth Census, Manufacturers*, p. 6 shows a shrinking between 1890 and 1900 from 1805 to 250 firms, while their value rose from $6 659 727 to $23 192 785.

40. See Weikel, 'Research as a Function of the Pharmaceutical Industry'.

41. In 1888 *Science* magazine published the results of a survey by an early bacteriologist, H. W. Conn, 'Bacteriology in our Medical Schools', *Science*, 11 (1888) pp. 123–6, about attitudes towards bacteriology in American medical schools. All the large medical colleges in the country were among the twenty-eight schools which responded. The sample included schools which educated about half of the doctors in the country. The response was mixed, all the more so since no distinction was drawn between the teaching of bacteriology and prevailing attitudes towards the germ theory of disease. Although only four respondents clearly opposed the germ theory, the return was 25 per cent, so one can assume that a large number of the smaller schools either found the survey of no interest, too much of a bother, or were opposed to any consideration of the germ theory or bacteriology. In general, however, a favourable view of bacteriology emerged from Conn's summary and it was apparent that many of the schools which did not already have laboratories intended to establish them. Ten colleges claimed to have laboratories suitable for teaching bacteriology and six other schools indicated that although they did not have a laboratory, the germ theory was taught. Of the Philadelphia medical schools, the three largest, the University of Pennsylvania, Hahnemann Medical College and Jefferson Medical College, all wrote that they had some facilities for laboratory instruction and intended to integrate bacteriology into their teaching of pathology. The 1888 survey showed that the three main areas in which bacteriology was taught were pathology, hygiene and surgery; and Philadelphia did not deviate from this pattern. Robert Koch's work was regarded in the United States, as in Germany, as the model for bacteriology. Two medical institutions noted in their replies to Conn that they followed

Koch in some way or other. The Medical College of Ohio boasted that it had 'a fully equipped bacteriology laboratory. The laboratory was furnished directly from Koch's laboratory in Berlin'. And at the Medical Department of the City of New York, 'a special instructor, a pupil of Koch, gives bacteriological instruction'.

42. George Rosen, *History of Public Health* (New York: M.D. Publications, 1958) p. 331.

43. On the impact of bacteriology on surgery in the United States, see Jonathan Liebenau, 'The Reception of Antisepsis in the United States', paper presented at the annual meeting, American Association for the History of Medicine, 12 May 1978; Gert Brieger, 'American Surgery and the Germ Theory of Disease', *Bulletin of the History of Medicine*, 39 (1965) pp. 135–45; Thomas Garipy, 'The Reception of Listerism in America', MA thesis, Notre Dame University, 1976; Phyllis A. Richmond, 'American Attitudes Toward the Germ Theory of Disease (1860–1880)', *Journal of the History of Medicine and Allied Sciences*, 9 (1954) pp. 428–54.

44. This was the attitude implicit in Conn, 'Bacteriology', and was the base on which the Johns Hopkins University Medical School built its reputation. Considering the difficulties involved in beginning bacteriological work and the continued resistance to it in the United States, one might well be surprised by the relatively favourable attitude towards bacteriology shown in the 1888 survey. A. Alexander Smith described the attitude he believed accounted for American receptivity to Koch: 'Scientific men had been prepared by the labors of earlier investigators to accept Koch's conclusions': 'Address in Medicine, the Practice of Medicine in the Light of Bacteriological Researches', *New York State Medical Association, Transactions*, 12 (1895) pp. 193–206. See also Rosen, *Public Health*, p. 332.

45. See, for example, Fielding H. Garrison, *An Introduction to the History of Medicine*, 4th ed. (Philadelphia: W. B. Saunders, 1929) Chap. 12.

46. H. Schadewaldt, 'Behring, Emil von', *Dictionary of Scientific Biography*, Vol. 1 (New York: Scribner, 1970–80), pp. 574–8 (henceforth *DSB*); Claude E. Dolman, 'Ehrlich, Paul', *DSB*, Vol. 4, pp. 295–305; Dolman, 'Koch, Heinrich Hermann Roberts', *DSB*, Vol. 7, pp. 420–35.

47. An interesting perception of the 'unbelievable skepticism' of American reaction to the work of Pasteur and Koch is presented by Joseph McFarland, 'The Beginning of Bacteriology in Philadelphia', *Bulletin of the History of Medicine*, 5 (1937) p. 151.

48. Garrison, *History of Medicine*, pp. 578–80; Dolman, 'Koch', *DSB*.

49. Ibid. Robert Koch, 'Zur Untersuchung von pathogenen Organismen', *Mittheilungen aus dem Kaiserlichen Gesundheitsamt*, 1 (1881) pp. 1–48.

50. Koch's articles on disinfection, such as that written with G. Wolfhuegel, 'Untersuchungen ueber die Disinfection mit heisser Luft', *Mittheilungen aus dem Kaiserlichen Gesundheitsamt* 1 (1881) pp. 301–21 were translated and abstracted in English.

51. George Washington Corner, *Two Centuries of Medicine. A History of the School of Medicine, University of Pennslyvania*, (Philadelphia: Lippin-

cott, 1965) p. 74.

52. Donald Fleming, *William H. Welch and the Rise of Modern Medicine* (Boston: Little, Brown, 1954).

53. Charles Edward A. Winslow, *The Life of Herman M. Biggs Physician and Statesman of the Public Health* (Philadelphia: Lea and Febiger, 1929).

54. Thomas N. Bonner, *American Doctors and German Universities. A Chapter in International Intellectual Relations, 1870–1914*, (Lincoln: University of Nebraska Press, 1963) pp. 30–40.

55. Ibid. See also Fleming, *Welch*; and Winslow, *Biggs*.

56. A third German bacteriological journal, the *Centralblatt fuer Bacteriologie und Parasitenkunden* was established in 1888.

57. *Annales de l'Institut Pasteur*, 1 (1888).

58. Edgar March Crookshank, *An Introduction to Practical Bacteriology, Based upon the Methods of Koch* (New York: J. H. Vail, 1886); E. M. Crookshank, *Manual of Bacteriology* (New York, J. H. Vail, 1887); and E. M. Crookshank, *A Textbook of Bacteriology* (London: Lewis, 1886 and Philadelphia: W. B. Saunders, 1897).

59. M. V. Ball, *Essentials of Bacteriology* (Philadelphia: W. B. Saunders, 1891). The first edition of Ball's text was written after the most cursory study of the subject. Ball had been a student of Jacob DeCosta's at Jefferson Medical College (MD 1889) where he attended guest lectures in bacteriology by the Berlin professor, Julius Salinger. Ball also travelled to Germany, visiting Koch, Behring and Fraenkel. See Joseph McFarland, 'The Beginning of Bacteriology', pp. 190–3.

60. McFarland, 'The Beginning of Bacteriology', pp. 157–8; see also p. 151.

61. Conn, 'Bacteriology'.

62. Corner, *Two Centuries of Medicine*, pp. 182–3; McFarland, 'The Beginning of Bacteriology', pp. 163–70.

63. Allen J. Smith, 'Bacillus Caruleus', *University Medical Magazine*, 1 (1888) pp. 43, 188. Laboratory note by H. F. Formad.

64. Charles K. Mills, 'The Philadelphia Almhouse and Philadelphia Hospital from 1854 to 1908', in John Welch Croskey (ed.) *History of Blockley. A History of the Philadelphia General Hospital, 1731 to 1928* (Philadelphia: F. A. Davis, 1929) p. 83; and Edward B. Krumbhaar, 'The History of Pathology at the Philadelphia General Hospital', *Medical Life*, 40 (1933) pp. 170–2. Formad had a medical degree from Heidelberg and immigrated to the United States in the 1870s. In 1880 at the age of thirty-three he was appointed 'microscopist' at the Blockley Hospital.

65. McFarland, 'Beginning of Bacteriology', pp. 154–5.

66. Ibid.

67. Ibid., pp. 155–6. See also David H. Bergey, 'Early Instruction in Bacteriology in the United States', *Annals of Medical History*, 1 (1917) pp. 426–7.

68. McFarland, 'Beginning of Bacteriology', p. 160.

69. John M. Swan, Notebook from course by Juan Guiteras, General Pathology 1890–91, in College of Physicians of Philadelphia. Swan's notes indicate extensive bacteriological teaching, but in 1893 McFarland was a student at the Medical School and had no such instruction at all:

McFarland, autobiographical notes, McFarland Papers. Guiteras had in fact scheduled a course in 'bacteriology' for the class following Swan's, but made a trip to his native Cuba that year to study cholera, so the course was cancelled. University of Pennsylvania, Catalogue 1890–91, in University of Pennsylvania Archives. See also McFarland, 'Beginning of Bacteriology', p. 160; also 'John Guiteras', *Dictionary of American Biography*.

70. McFarland, Vita, McFarland Papers.
71. McFarland, 'Beginning of Bacteriology', pp. 170–2.
72. Ibid.
73. Corner, *Two Centuries of Medicine*, pp. 182–3; McFarland, 'Beginning of Bacteriology', pp. 163–9.
74. University of Pennsylvania, Catalogue 1895, in University of Pennsylvania Archives.
75. Ibid.
76. John Shaw Billings, 'The Objectives, Plans and Needs of the Laboratory of Hygiene. An Address Delivered at the Opening of the Laboratory of Hygiene of the University of Pennsylvania, February 22, 1896', *Medical News* (Philadelphia) 60 (1892) pp. 232–5.
77. University of Pennsylvania, Catalogue 1895.
78. Ibid.; see also McFarland, 'Beginning of Bacteriology', p. 165.
79. Ibid.
80. Ibid. Fielding H. Garrison, *John Shaw Billings, A Memoir* (New York: G. P. Putnam, 1915).
81. Alexander C. Abbott, *The Hygiene of Transmissible Diseases* (Philadelphia: Lea Brothers, 1909).
82. Benjamin Lee, Opening exercises, Laboratory of Hygiene, University of Pennsylvania Archives.
83. When advertising to physicians, in particular, companies such as Parke Davis, Smith Kline, Wyeth and others stressed their links with academic science. These links usually proved tenuous. As, for example, the claim made by Smith Kline that Mr J. William Landis and Professor F. G. Ryan of the Philadelphia College of Pharmacy worked in the company laboratory, made in an advertisement run in the *Pharmaceutical Record* (1891) p. 10.
84. Smith Kline and French, 'Analytical Laboratory Notes', SmithKline Records. See also photographs of the laboratory and laboratory workers in the photograph collection.
85. Ibid.
86. For the links between Parke Davis and the University of Michigan see Steckl, 'Biological Standardization', and Weikel, 'Research as a Function of the Pharmaceutical Industry'; also Parke Davis, *Parke Davis at 100*.
87. Smith Kline, 'Analytical Laboratory Notes', p. 7.
88. 'Smith Kline', *Pharmaceutical Era*, p. 956.
89. Ibid.; also Smith Kline, 'Analytical Laboratory Notes'.
90. See Joseph England File; Giant Chemical Company File, SmithKline Records.
91. Marion, *SmithKline*.

92. Smith Kline, 'Analytical Laboratory Notes'.
93. Ibid.; see also George R. Pancoast File, SmithKline Records.
94. Ibid.
95. Kahn, *Eli Lilly*, pp. 25–6.
96. Joseph England, *The First Hundred Years of the Philadelphia College of Pharmacy* (Philadelphia: Philadelphia College of Pharmacy, 1921). See also Kahn, *Eli Lilly*.
97. Kahn, *Eli Lilly*, p. 27.
98. Ibid.
99. Ibid., p. 73.
100. Steckl, 'Biological Standardization', p. 10; Albert B. Lyons, *Manual of Practical Pharmaceutical Assaying* (Detroit: Parke Davis and Company, 1886); Wilber L. Schoville, 'Our Honorary President, Albert Brown Lyons, A.M., M.D., F.R.C.S.', *Journal of the American Pharmaceutical Association*, 2 (1913) p. 1579.
101. Parke, Davis and Company, *Scientific Contributions from the Laboratories 1866–1966* (Detroit: Parke Davis, 1966).
102. Schoville, 'Lyons'. Parke Davis was more restrained than their competitors in exploiting scientific credentials in this early period.
103. Weikel, 'Research as a Function of the Pharmaceutical Industry', p. 35.
104. Schoville, 'Lyons'.
105. Lyons, *Manual*, p. 1.
106. 'Lyman Kebler', *American Men of Science (AMS)*, 5 (1925).
107. Smith Kline, 'Analytical Laboratory Notes'; also prominently featured in advertisements; SmithKline Records and collections at the College of Physicians and Smithsonian Institution.
108. Ibid. Also England, *Philadelphia College of Physicians*.
109. Ibid. 'Lyman Kebler' *AMS*; Oscar E. Anderson, *Health of A Nation: Harvey W. Wiley's Fight for Pure Foods* (New York: Norton, 1958).
110. *The Druggists' Bulletin*, 1 (1887) title page.
111. Thomas Mahoney, *The Merchants of Life. An Account of the American Pharmaceutical Industry* (New York: Harper, 1959) p. 71.
112. Ibid., p. 72. Taylor, 'Forty-Five Years', pp. 472–3.
113. Henry H. Rustby, *Jungle Memories* (New York: Whittlesey House, 1933).
114. Rustby's book became popular in the 'boys' adventure' genre.
115. Taylor, 'Forty-Five Years'.
116. *The Pharmacopoeia of the United States of America* began in 1820 (first edition Easton, Pennsylvania). Two revisions were issued in 1830, one from Philadelphia, the other from New York. Later editions were issued in 1840, 1850, etc., up to the present. See also Martin Inventius Wilbert, *Changes in the Pharmacopoeia and the National Formulary* (Washington, DC: USGPO, 1917). The *National Formulary*, 1st ed. (Washington, DC: American Pharmaceutical Association, 1888) listed 'unofficial preparations'. It appeared in 1896, 1906, 1916, etc.
117. Parke, Davis and Company, *Organic Materia Medica* (Detroit: Parke, Davis, 1890) p. iv; (1st ed., 1890).
118. Kahn, *Eli Lilly*, p. 27.
119. Robert B. Shaw, *History of the Comstock Patent Medicine Business and*

Dr. Morse's Indian Root Pills (Washington, DC: Smithsonian Institution Press, 1972). See also James Harvey Young, *The Toadstool Millionaires: A Social History of Patent Medicines in America Before Federal Regulation* (Princeton: Princeton University Press, 1961).

CHAPTER 4

1. See H. J. Parish, *A History of Immunization* (Edinburgh: Livingstone, 1965) pp. 118–40; F. W. Andrews *et al.*, *Diphtheria. Its Bacteriology, Pathology and Immunology* (London: HMSO, 1923) pp. 126–9.
2. Chart in *Phildelphia Bureau of Health, Annual Report for 1918* (Philadelphia, 1919) p. 151. Before 1899 the Bureau was named the Board of Health.
3. *Philadelphia Bureau of Health, Annual Reports* (1880–1920). See especially *Annual Report* (1895) p. 186.
4. Andrews *et al.*, *Diptheria*, pp. 13*ff*.
5. Ibid.; Pierre Fidele Bretonneau, *Des Inflammations Speciales du tissu Muqueux, et en particular de la Diptherite, ou Inflammation Pelliculaire* (Paris: Crevot, 1826).
6. *Philadelphia Bureau of Health, Annual Reports* (1880–1920); William H. Park and W. L. Beebe, 'Diptheria and Pseudo-Diptheria, a report to Hermann M. Biggs . . . on the bacteriological examination of 5,611 cases . . .', *Medical Record*, 46 (1894) p. 385.
7. For a graphic description of the effects of diptheria on children, see 'Sir Charles Sherrington's First Use of Diptheria Antitoxin Made in England', *Notes and Records of the Royal Society of London*, 4 (1946) p. 156–9; also Sinclair Lewis, *Martin Arrowsmith* (London: Jonathan Cape, 1925); Wayde W. Oliver, *The Man Who Lived for Tomorrow. A Biography of William Hallock Park* (New York: Dutton, 1941) p. 85; for a contemporary description, see Edwin O. Jordan, *A Text-Book of General Bacteriology* (Philadelphia: W. B. Saunders, 1908) pp. 229–31.
8. US Bureau of the Census, *Historical Statistics of the United States, from Colonial Times to the Present* (Washington, DC: USGPO, 1976) p. 58; *New York City Board of Health Annual Reports* (1890–1930); *Philadelphia Annual Reports* (1890–1930).
9. Wayland Hand, 'Folk Medicine', paper presented at the Smithsonian Institution, March 1980.
10. Laryngectomy and intubation were commonly used for more severe cases, see Edwin Rosenthal, 'Reduced Period of Intubation by the Serum Treatment of Laryngeal Diptheria', *Pennsylvania Medical Society, Transactions*, 27 (1896) pp. 238–50; and E. Rosenthal, 'A Report of 100 Cases of Diptheria of the Larynx Treated by Intubation', *Medical Bulletin* (September and October 1894).
11. The diptheria ward at Blockley was opened in 1893, see William M. Welch, 'The Municipal Hospital for Contagious and Infectious Diseases',

in Frederick P. Henry, *Founder's Week Memorial Volume* (Philadelphia: City of Philadelphia, 1909) pp. 546–54; also A. C. Abbott, 'The Development of Public Health Work in Philadelphia', in ibid., pp. 563–92. See also Charles K. Mills, 'The Philadelphia Almshouse and the Philadelphia Hospital from 1854 to 1901', in John Welsh Croskey (ed.) *History of Blockley, A History of the Philadelphia General Hospital from its Inception 1731–1928* (Philadelphia: Blockley Hospital, 1929) p. 94.

12. William Bulloch, *The History of Bacteriology* (New York: Dover, 1979) p. 237; F. Loeffler, 'Untersuchungen ueber die Bedeutung der Mikroorganismen fuer die Entstehung der Diphtherie beim Menschen, bei der Taube und beim Kalbe', *Mittheilungen aus dem Kaiserlichen Gesundscheitsamt*, 2 (1884) pp. 421–99.

13. E. Klebs, 'Ueber Diptherie', *Verhandlung d. Congress f. innere Medizin* (Wiesbaden) 43 (1883) p. 139; Bernhard Moellers, *Robert Koch, Persoenlichkeit und Lebenswerk, 1843–1910* (Hannover: Schmoll, 1950) pp. 527–32.

14. H. Zeiss and R. Beiling, *Behring, Gestalt und Werk* (Berlin: Schultz, 1941) pp. 54ff, 106, 248. See also Hoechst, Dokumente aus Hoechster Archiven, *Behring* (Frankfurt: Hoechst, 1967).

15. Zeiss and Bieling, *Behring*, pp. 58–61.

16. E. Behring and S. Kitasato, 'Ueber das Zustandekommen der Diphtherie-Immunitaet und der Tetanus-Immunitaet bei Thieren', *Deutsche Medicinische Wochenschrift*, 16 (1890) p. 1113.

17. E. Behring, 'Weitere Bemerkungen zur Diphtherieheilungsfrage', *Deutsche Medicinische Wochenschrift*, 20 (1894) p. 645; E. Behring, 'Zur Diphtherieimmunisirungsfrage', ibid., 20 (1894) p. 865; Zeiss and Bieling, *Behring*, p. 113.

18. E. Roux and A. Yersin, 'Contribution a l'étude de la diphtherie', *Annales de l'Institut Pasteur*, 2 (1888) p. 629; ibid., 3 (1889) p. 273; ibid., 4 (1890) p. 385; E. Roux and L. Villare, 'Contribution a l'étude dui tetanos, prevention et traitment par le serum antitoxique', *Annales de l'Institut Pasteur*, 7 (1893) p. 65; E. Roux and L. Martin, 'Contribution a l'étude de la diphtherie (serum-therapie)', *Annales de l'Institut Pasteur*, 8 (1894) p. 609; Emile Lagrance, *Monsieur Roux* (Brussels: Goemaere, 1954) pp. 119–23.

19. E. Roux, L. Martin and A. Chaillou, 'Trois cents cas de diphtherie traites par les serum antidiphtherique', *Annales de l'Institut Pasteur*, 8 (1894) p. 640; Lagrance, *Roux*, pp. 143–5.

20. Emile Roux, 'Sur les serums antitoxiques', *Cong. Internat. d'hyg. et de Demog. c. r., 1894 Budapesth*, 2 (1896) p. 27; 'Sur la serum therapie de la diphtherie', ibid., p. 188.

21. Lagrange, *Roux*, pp. 153–4.

22. J. Liebenau, 'Patents in the Chemical Industry', in J. Liebenau (ed.) *The Challenge of New Technology* (London: Gower, 1987).

23. Rene Vallery-Radot, *The Life of Pasteur*, Vol. II (London: Constable, 1902) pp. 303–7.

24. Kinyoun, 'Report', in *United States Marine Hospital and Public Health Service, Annual Reports* (Washington, DC: USGPO, 1895).

25. Ibid. There were significant problems with large-scale production. For

example, the pH level was not specified and proper aeration and mixing was not defined.

26. Hygienic Laboratory Records, National Archives; The Smithsonian Institution has one of the early bottles of antitoxin produced at the laboratory, dated 1895.
27. Oliver, *Park*; David Blancher, 'Workshops of the Bacteriological Revolution: A History of the Laboratories of the New York City Department of Health, 1892–1912', PhD dissertation, City University of New York, 1979. In 1894 Henry Walcott organised a laboratory to produce diphtheria antitoxin for use in the state of Massachusetts; Dr J. L. Goodale was appointed to set up the laboratory, and Theobald Smith assigned to the position of director for the next year. See B. C. Rosenkrantz, *Public Health and the State. Changing Views in Massachusetts 1842–1936* (Cambridge, Mass.: Harvard University Press, 1972) p. 113.
28. S. P. Reismann, 'Joseph McFarland', *Transactions and Studies of the College of Physicians of Philadelphia*, 3rd series (1939) pp. 133–5.
29. Vita, McFarland Papers, College of Physicians of Philadelphia.
30. The Board had inadequate resources from the beginning and used both the stables of the Fire Department and the Police Department during 1894–96. See Minutes, 1895 and J. J. McFarland, 'The Beginning of Bacteriology in Philadelphia', *Bulletin of the History of Medicine*, 5 (1935) pp. 182–3.
31. Croskey, *Blockley*, p. 85.
32. John Thomas Mahoney, *The Merchants of Life. A History of Pharmaceutical Manufacturing in the United States* (New York: Harper, 1959) p. 163; *Philadelphia Bureau of Health, Annual Report* (1910), p. 462–3.
33. See following papers in *Journal of the American Medical Association*, 27 (1896): J. Fletcher Ingals, 'Orrhotherapy in Diphtheria', pp. 1–4; Charles T. McClintock, 'The Outlook in Serum Therapy', pp. 4–7; E. L. Larkins, 'The Use of Antitoxin in the Treatment of Diphtheria and Membraneous Croup; With a Collective Report of One Hundred and Thirty-two Cases', pp. 7–10; Edwin Rosenthal, 'Serum Therapy in Diphtheria', pp. 11–14; Harold C. Ernst, 'An Introduction to the Discussion Upon "Blood-Serum Therapeutics"', pp. 14–17; Elmer Lee, 'The Fallacy of Antitoxin Treatment as a Cure for Diphtheria', pp. 17–19; Louis Fischer, 'Some Practical Points on the Combined Effects of Antitoxin and Intubation, with Special Reference to Infant Feeding in Malignant Diphtheria', pp. 19–20; Joseph William Stickler, 'An Experience with Antitoxin with Instructive Results', ibid., pp 20–21; 'Discussion on Papers of Drs Elmer Lee, Joseph W. Stickler and Louis Fischer', Edwin Klebs, W. E. Casselberry, Dr Ross, Dr Thomason, Dr Larrabee, W. J. Bell, H. E. Garrison, Dr Vaker, Dr Hodges, D. C. Wilson, Dr Knipe, Elmer Lee, W. A. Dixon, ibid., pp. 21–6; B. Meade Bolton, 'Theory of Serum Therapy; Contribution from the Bacteriologic Laboratory of the City of Philadelphia', ibid., pp. 26–27; W. P. Northrup, Joseph O'Dwyer, Samuel S. Adams, Committee members, 'Report of the American Pediatric Society's Collective Investigation into the Use of Antitoxin in the Treatment of Diphtheria in Private Practice', ibid., pp. 27–35. See also J. Fletcher Ingals, 'Correspondence – Orrhotherapy in Diphtheria', ibid., p. 49; and P. M. Bracelin, 'Corres-

pondence – The Bracelin Remedy in Diphtheria', ibid., pp. 49–50.
34. *Philadelphia Annual Reports* (1897–1900); Rosenkrantz, *Public Health*, pp. 113–14, 124–6.
35. Emil Behring, 'Untersuchungen ueber das Zustandekommen der Diphtherie – Immunitaet bei Thieren', *Deutsche Medicinische Wochenschrift*, 16 (1890) p. 1145.
36. Oliver, *Park*; W. H. Park and A. W. Williams, 'The Production of Diphtheria Toxin', *Journal of Experimental Medicine*, 1 (1896) p. 164.
37. Oliver, *Park*; Blancher, 'Workshop'.
38. McFarland, 'Beginning of Bacteriology'.
39. *Philadelphia Annual Reports* (1896–1906).
40. *Philadelphia Annual Report* (1910) p. 22.
41. Rosenkrantz, *Public Health*, p. 123.
42. H. K. Mulford Company, *Price List* (1900).
43. Mahoney, *Merchants of Life*, p. 462.

CHAPTER 5

1. In Philadelphia the Department of Public Health dispensed 900 000 units of diphtheria antitoxin in 1896, 8 061 000 in 1901, and 34 000 000 in 1906. *Philadelphia Board of Health Annual Report* (1906) p. 18.
2. Commonwealth of Pennsylvania, 'Report on the Vaccine Farms and Antitoxin Propagating Establishments of the United States, and their Products, and on Certain Imported Antitoxins', *Twelfth Annual Report of the State Board of Health* (1897) pp. 153–211.
3. *New York City Board of Health, Annual Reports* (1893–1900).
4. Wayde Oliver, *The Man Who Lived for Tomorrow. William Hallock Park* (New York: Dutton, 1941).
5. Francis E. Stewart, [Mulford Company History] 'Twenty Years, 1891–1911', 1911, Mulford Company Records, Merck and Company Archives, West Point, Pennsylvania. The Mulford Company Records collection will hereafter be referred to as Mulford Records.
6. H. K. Mulford Company, *Price List* (Philadelphia: Mulford, n.d. [c. 1893]) Mulford Records.
7. US Patent No. 413 310, 22 October, 1889. Shown in the 1893 *Price List*; see also Stewart, 'Twenty Years'. Earlier patents for fast-acting tablet machines were filed on behalf of Wyeth Brothers, No. 215 452, 28 March, 1879, to J. H. Gill assigned to Henry Bower (of Wyeth), and No. 323 349 to John Lusby in 1885. See also file 'Wyeth History', in Wyeth Papers.
8. US Patent No. 413 310, Oberlin Smith was probably the actual inventor; Henry Mulford was possibly included to simplify the assignation of the patent rights. He may have helped in the development of the machine in its earlier stages.
9. F. E. Stewart, 'Mulford Growth Shows Great Achievement', *Northwestern Druggist*, 30 (1922) p. 14. This machine, together with an improvement of 1897, became a popular item which the company sold for

$100 for a hand-operated model, and $200 for a power-driven model. H. K. Mulford Company, *Price List* (Philadelphia: Mulford, 1900) p. 568. The improvements were made by Abraham Rowland Morris, patented and assigned to Mulford in 1899, US Patent No. 617 255, 3 January, 1899.

10. Editorial, *Practical Therapeutics* (February 1898) p. 1 quoted in the *Price List* (1900) p. 526.
11. Ibid.
12. Some price lists, such as the extensive one of 1900, marked 'the most popular prescriptions' on every page. Those named here all received two stars.
13. *Price List* (1900) p. 535.
14. Ibid., p. 532.
15. *Price List* (1893).
16. *Price List* (1900).
17. H. E. Ditzel, 'Memorandum: History of the H. K. Mulford Company', 13 March 1963, p. 5, Mulford Records.
18. *Price List* (1893).
19. H. K. Mulford Company, '25th Anniversary Souvenir', 1916, Mulford Records.
20. Stewart, 'Twenty Years'.
21. Joseph McFarland, 'The Beginning of Bacteriology in Philadelphia', *Bulletin of the History of Medicine*, 5 (1937) pp. 188–9. This marvellous recollection by McFarland, then the retired Professor of Pathology at the University of Pennsylvania, contains lively anecdotes about his years at Mulford from 1894 to 1896.
22. Ibid.; antivenom experiments were continuously done at Mulford as part of a general investigation of toxicology. In 1927 the company formed the American Antivenom Institute as one means of promoting their long line of snakebite remedies. *Bulletin of the American Antivenom Institute*, 1 (1927).
23. McFarland, 'Beginning of Bacteriology', p. 184. The bacteriologist's salary at the Bureau of Health was fixed on 27 February 1895, see *Philadelphia Board of Health, Annual Report for 1895* (1896) p. 317.
24. One recognition of McFarland's success at the company was given when, in 1899, McFarland Hall was opened as a new biological laboratory. H. K. Mulford Company, 'Guide Book, Mulford Biological Laboratories', n.d. [c. 1935], Mulford Records.
25. 'Personnel file, Henry K. Mulford', Mulford Records. Obituary, 'Henry K. Mulford', *Northwestern Druggist*, 45 (1937) pp. 59–60. On Milton Campbell, see Stewart, 'Mulford Growth'.
26. File, 'Diphtheria Antitoxic Serum', Mulford Records. Fischer's more extensive report appeared in the *Medical Record*, 6 October 1894, and was noted in a running bibliography kept at the company.
27. McFarland, 'Beginning of Bacteriology', pp. 181–4.
28. Ibid., p. 184. McFarland himself records that 'after mature deliberation and definite understandings regarding many things, I agreed to accept'.
29. Stewart, 'Mulford Growth'.
30. Peter Steckl, 'Biological Standardization of Drugs Before 1928', PhD dissertation, University of Wisconsin, 1969, pp. 64–5.

31. Both claims were repeatedly made in advertising and there is certainly no clear answer to the question of who might have been the first to market the product, though McFarland maintained many years later that Mulford was first. This claim followed his break with the company in 1896 and a period as an employee of Parke Davis. See Ditzel, 'Memorandum', where McFarland is quoted.
32. H. K. Mulford Company, 'The Present Status of Diphtheria Antitoxin', (advertisement) 1895, Mulford Records.
33. Pearson (1868–1909) was much appreciated by the company, which named him frequently in advertisements. See, for example, Mulford, 'The Present Status'.
34. Ibid.; H. K. Mulford Company, 'The Antitoxin Treatment of Diphtheria with Bibliography, Official Reports and Clinical Notes' (advertisement) 1896, Mulford Records; McFarland, 'Beginning of Bacteriology'.
35. McFarland, 'Beginning of Bacteriology', p. 186.
36. H. K. Mulford Company, 'The Present Status of Diphtheria Antitoxic Serum' (advertisement) c. late 1897 or early 1898, Library of the College of Physicians of Philadelphia.
37. Philadelphia Bureau of Health, 'Minutes', 7 November 1894. Antitoxin was ordered from Behring in November. Stewart, 'Twenty Years'.
38. McFarland, 'Beginning of Bacteriology', p. 187. Also Mulford, 'Present Status', (1895).
39. 'Personnel file, Henry K. Mulford'.
40. Bergey reappeared as Henry Mulford's Director of Research in Biology for National Drug Company, a firm Mulford established with his son after the H. K. Mulford Company merged with Sharpe and Dohme in 1929.
41. H. K. Mulford Company, 'Diphtheria Antitoxic Serum, Announcement', 1895, Mulford Records.
42. Laboratory of Hygiene Records, University of Pennsylvania Archives; file, 'Mulford History', Mulford Records.
43. File, 'Diphtheria Antitoxin', Mulford Records.
44. Some homeopaths argued that antitoxins ought to be accepted on the grounds that they could be reconciled with the principles of like-cures dilution. See, for example, Joseph McFarland, 'The Efficiency of Antitoxin as a Remedial Agent in Diphtheria', *Pennsylvania State Board of Health, Annual Report* (1896) pp. 621–6.
45. Fielding H. Garrison, *An Introduction to the History of Medicine*, 4th ed. (Philadelphia: Saunders, 1929) p. 438.
46. Two conferences were held in 1896 to promote this idea, one sponsored by the Pennsylvania Board of Health, the other at the American Medical Association convention in Atlanta.
47. Emil Behring and Shibasaburo Kitasato, 'Ueber das Zustandekommen der Diphtherie-Immunitaet und der Tetanus-Immunitaet bei Thieren', *Deutsche Medicinische Wochenschrift*, 16 (1890) pp. 1113–14, 1145–48.
48. Tetanus antitoxin was available by 1895 and was listed in advertisements from that year. See 'Advertisements', Mulford Records.
49. Editorial, *Keystone*, 1, 22 November 1918, p. 1. *Keystone*, the company newsletter, appeared irregularly as a short (often four pages) gossip

sheet, social calendar and general interest paper. It fostered a company identity among workers and explained some policy decisions made by the Board of Directors. Occasionally articles relating to the history of a company department appeared and the scientific staff sometimes wrote about their work.

50. *Keystone*, 1, 1 January 1919, p. 1.
51. Ibid. Laboratory records in the Merck archives are closed by a company policy protecting trade secrets, but they do show attempts to produce antitoxins from all culturable pathogens.
52. The distinction was made between bacteria which give off exotoxins which allow the production of antitoxins and those which do not. Mulford produced a long line of 'bacterins' made from killed bacteria rather than toxins from them.
53. The production of bacterins followed the same procedure as antitoxins.
54. Mulford, *Price List*, 1898.
55. M. J. Rosenau, *The Immunity Unit for Standardizing Diphtheria Antitoxin*, Hygienic Laboratory Bulletin No. 21 (Washington DC: USGPO, 1905) pp. 18–24.
56. P. Ehrlich, 'Die Wertbemessung des diphtherieheilserums and deren theoretische grundlagen', *Klinische jahrbuch* (Jena) 6 (1897) pp. 299–376. On Ehrlich see R. Otto and H. Hetsch, 'Die Pruefung und Wertbemessung der Sera und Impfstoffe', in W. Kolle (ed.) *Arbeiten aus den Staatsinstitut fuer Experimentelle Therapie und der Georg Speyer-Hause zu Frankfurt a. M.,* part 19 (Jena: Georg Speyer-Haus, 1927). Mulford, 'Diphtheria Antitoxic Serum', p. 19.
57. Mulford, *Price List*, 1900, p. 569; Edwin Rosenthal, 'Diphtheria Antitoxin', *Philadelphia College of Pharmacy, Alumni Report*, 33 (1900) p. 32.
58. Mulford, 'Diphtheria Antitoxic Serum', p. 19.
59. Stewart, 'Mulford Growth', p. 14.
60. Mulford, 'Advertisements', Mulford Records; Parke Davis, 'Trade Catalogue', Division of Medical Science, National Museum of American History, Smithsonian Institution, Washington, DC. This latter collection will be referred to as Smithsonian. See also Steckl, 'Biological Standardization', pp. 113 *ff.*
61. Mulford, *Price List*, 1900, p. 570.
62. Quoted in ibid.
63. Stewart, 'Mulford Growth'; Ditzel, 'Memorandum', p. 1.
64. Editorial, *Mulford Digest*, I (1912) p. 2.
65. Ditzel, 'Memorandum'.
66. Ibid.
67. Ibid. See also Stewart, 'Mulford Growth'.
68. This statement appeared in most advertising after 1900.
69. Compare, for example, the earlier statement that the company did not seek monopoly 'obtained either by secret formulas or process or product patents', (1900) with a price list from c. 1923: '. . . obtained by secret formulas'.
70. Stewart, 'Twenty Years'.
71. Mulford, *Price List*, 1912, Mulford Records, p. 20.

72. This was an underlying theme to their advertisements to physicians.
73. Mulford, 'Advertisements'.
74. Mulford, 'Guide Book'.
75. Stewart, 'Twenty Years', p. 9.
76. Mulford, *Price List*, 1900, p. 570.
77. Ibid.
78. Ibid.
79. Ibid.
80. Ibid.
81. Ibid., p. 572.
82. 'Report', *Pennsylvania State Board of Health, Annual Report* (1897) pp. 208–10.
83. Ibid.
84. Ibid.
85. 'Inspections', US Hygienic Laboratory Records, National Archives.
86. Photographs, Mulford Records.
87. Mulford, 'Diphtheria Antitoxic Serum', 1902, p. 17.
88. Ibid., p. 19.
89. Photographs, Mulford Records: Mulford, *Price List*, 1900, p. 574; see also *Philadelphia College of Pharmacy, Alummi Report*, December 1899, p. 258.
90. Walter Brooks and Robert C. Purcel, 'A Trip to the Vaccine Farm of the H. K. Mulford Company', *Philadelphia College of Pharmacy, Alummi Report*, December 1899, p. 252.
91. This was one of the main purposes of the company newsletter, *Keystone*.
92. 'Retirement of Miss Corsi', *Keystone*, 2 (1919) p. 6.
93. Mulford, *Price List*, 1900, p. 574.
94. Ibid., p. 575.
95. Photographs, Mulford Records.
96. 'Advertisements', Mulford Records.
97. Mulford, *Price Lists*, (1893–1927).
98. Stewart, 'Twenty Years'. pp. 6–9.
99. Taken from publicity of the Syracuse (New York) Department of Public Safety and quoted in Mulford, 'Diphtheria Antitoxic Serum', 1902.
100. Stewart, 'Mulford Growth', p. 13.
101. Ibid., p. 14.
102. Mulford, 'Diphtheria Antitoxic Serum', 1896.
103. Mulford, 'Diphtheria Antitoxic Serum', 1905, in Library of the College of Physicians of Philadelphia.
104. Mulford, *Price List*, c. 1914, Mulford Records.
105. Mulford, 'Diphtheria Antitoxic Serum', 1902.
106. Wall chart, 1 September 1916, in Mulford Records.
107. Mulford also published a *Veterinary Bulletin* starting in 1915, also mimicking scholarly journals.
108. A. Parker Hitchens, 'The Treatment of Simple Catarrh of the Respiratory Passages with Bacterial Vaccines', *Medical Record*, 1 (1912) pp. 104–8.
109. Charles E. Vanderkleed (Chief Chemist, H. K. Mulford Company), 'Chemical and Physiological Standardization', address before the

Alumni of New York College of Pharmacy, and Frances E. Stewart, 'What is Meant by Drug Standardization', paper read to the annual meeting, National Dental Association, Mulford Records. See also: E. D. Reed and Charles E. Vanderkleed, 'The Standardization of Preparations of Digitalis by Physiological and Chemical Means', *American Journal of Pharmacology*, 80 (1908) p. 110; Charles E. Vanderkleed and L. Henry Bernegau, 'Can Uniform and Therefore "Standardized" Tinctures be Prepared from Assayed Drugs Without Assaying the Finished Product?', *Pennsylvania Pharmacological Association, Proceedings* (1908) pp. 176–80 (reprinted as a Mulford pamphlet) Mulford Records; H. K. Mulford Company, 'Importance of Digitalis Standardization', 1909, Mulford Records; Treasury Department, Public Health and Marine Hospital Service of the United States, Hygienic Laboratory, Bulletin No. 48, Charles Wallis Edmonds and Worth Hale, 'The Physiological Standardization of Digitalis', 1908; Charles C. Haskell, 'Physiological Methods for the Standardization of Digitalis', *American Journal of Pharmacy*, 83 (1911) p. 201 (Haskell worked for the Eli Lilly Company).

110. *Mulford Working Bulletin*, No. 6, 'Typho-Bacterin and Typho-Bacterin Mixed', revised edition of 1913 at the National Library of Medicine, Washington, DC.
111. *Keystone*, 2, 8 September 1919, p. 3.
112. Advertisement in *Philadelphia College of Pharmacy, Alumni Report*, 1900.
113. Ibid., 1894–1900; Parke Davis and Company, *Price List*, 1895; see also Steckl, 'Standardization', pp. 110–11.
114. Parke Davis and Company, 'A Souvenir of Parke Davis and Company', c. 1915, p. 30, Smithsonian. See also Steckl, 'Standardization', p. 10.
115. E. Rosenthal, 'Serum Therapy in Diphtheria', *Journal of the American Medical Association*, 27 (1896) pp. 11–14.
116. Ibid.
117. Ibid.
118. Oliver, *Park*; Barbara Gutmann Rosenkrantz, *Public Health and the State. Changing Views in Massachusetts, 1842–1936* (Cambridge, Mass.: Harvard University Press, 1972) pp. 113–14.
119. For a list of states which provided antitoxin free, see Herbert W. Conn, *Text-Book of Bacteriology* (Philadelphia: Saunders, 1902).
120. Rosenkrantz, *Public Health*, pp. 123–4.
121. John Thomas Mahoney, *The Merchants of Life. A History of Pharmaceutical Manufacturing in the United States* (New York: Harper, 1959) p. 162.
122. Ibid.
123. Minutes of Executive Meeting, 26 September 1918, Mulford Records.
124. H. K. Mulford Company, *Working Bulletin*, No. 6, p. 32.
125. Stewart, 'Mulford Growth', p. 15. See also Milton Campbell personnel file, Mulford Records.
126. H. K. Mulford Company, '"Vaccination" in Cancer. A Report of the Results of the Vaccination Therapy as Applied in 79 Cases of Human Cancer', *Mulford Digest*, 1 (1913) pp. 96–103.
127. Mulford, *Price List*, 1900, p. 538.

128. Ibid., p. 545.
129. 'Chats from the Laboratory', *Keystone*, 2 (1919) p. 8.
130. Edwin Rosenthal, 'Reduced Period of Intubation by the Serum Treatment of Laryngeal Diphtheria', *Pennsylvania Medical Society, Transactions*, 26 (1896) pp. 238–50.
131. W. F. Elgin, 'A Quarter Century of Vaccine Production with H. K. Mulford and Company', paper read at the C and C Club, 10 December 1923, Mulford Records. McFarland was also 'rewarded' with four months' absence on full pay to visit European laboratories in the summer of 1895; see McFarland, 'Beginning of Bacteriology', p. 183. *Pennsylvania State Board of Health, Annual Report* (1897) p. 206.
132. Stewart, 'Mulford Growth', p. 17.
133. Joseph W. England (ed.) *The First Century of the Philadelphia College of Pharmacy 1821–1921* (Philadelphia: Philadelphia College of Pharmacy, 1922).
134. *Keystone*, 2 (1919) p. 3.
135. This arrangement in 1917 pre-dated by ten years a similar contract between the University of Toronto and Eli Lilly for the production of insulin. See H. K. Mulford Company, 'Tethelin' (advertisement) c. 1918, Mulford Records.
136. Editorial, *Mulford Digest*, 1 (1912) p. 1.
137. Mulford, *Price List*, 1900, p. 569.
138. Mulford, 'Diphtheria Antitoxic Serum', 1902.
139. H. K. Mulford Company, 'The Complete Hay Fever Service', (advertisement), Mulford Records.
140. John Parascandola, 'The Rise of Pharmacology', unpublished paper, University of Wisconsin, 1979.
141. George M. Gould, 'Editorial', *Mulford Digest*, 1 (1912) p. 2.
142. Ibid.
143. Selman Waksman, *My Life With the Microbes* (London: The Scientific Book Club, 1958) pp. 89–90.
144. Ibid.
145. Mulford, *Price List*, 1900, p. 573.
146. Executive Committee Minutes, 8 November 1917.
147. Rosenau, *Standardizing Diphtheria Antitoxin*, p. 21.
148. Mulford, 'Diphtheria Antitoxin Serum', 1902.
149. See, for example, advertisements in *Philadelphia College of Pharmacy, Alumni Report* (1901–08).
150. Lederle seems to have been the most successful in securing contracts from big city departments. In 1907 it made substantial sales to the state boards of health in Ohio, Minnesota, Kentucky, Maryland, Illinois and a little to Rhode Island. US Hygienic Laboratory Records, National Archives, Box 340.
151. Hygienic Laboratory Records, National Archives, Box 340.
152. Dr J. H. Brown, interview August 1979, Marietta, Pennsylvania.
153. 'List of Biological Products', in *Working Bulletins*, Mulford Papers.
154. In 1905 Simon Flexner began a series of experiments at the Rockefeller Institute with a serum he devised with toxin from meningococcic cultures. Following the procedure for diphtheria antitoxin of injecting

horses and separating and concentrating the serum, he tested the product in 1905–06 on the full range of experimental animals and in 1908–09 on humans. *Journal of the American Medical Association* (1906ii) p. 560; (1909ii) p. 1143.

155. *Working Bulletin*, No. 8, 'Antimeningitis Serum', 1st ed., c. 1910.
156. Ibid.
157. 'Antimeningitis Serum' (advertisement) c. 1915, Mulford Papers.
158. A second edition of *Working Bulletin*, No. 8 was offered in 1917, advertising improvements in the serum and giving updated information on the treatment of meningitis: 'After a thorough study of all the well-known procedures with their complicated details, means have been evolved in the Mulford Laboratories by which the most advanced methods of treating cerebrospinal fever may be simplified and thus placed at the disposal of the physician', p. 1.
159. Ibid., p. 3.
160. Ibid.
161. Ibid., p. 9.
162. Ibid., back page.
163. Groesbeck Walsh, 'Fatility Rates in Cerebrospinal Meningitis', *Journal of the American Medical Association*, 110 (1938) pp. 1894–1896.
164. J. R. Grubb, 'Glenolden Then and Now, Business Methods in Biological Production', *Keystone*, 2 (1919) p. 2; Minutes of the Executive Meeting, 4 November 1918, Mulford Papers.
165. Minutes of the Executive Meeting, 11 November 1918.

CHAPTER 6

1. William M. Welch, 'The Discovery of Vaccination, and its Introduction into America', *Philadelphia College of Pharmacy, Alumni Report* (1897) pp. 51–62.
2. Two large vaccine companies, H. M. Alexander and Parke Davis were producing significant quantities of smallpox vaccine by the mid-1880s; local production had been done for some years previously.
3. The standard technique, using 'dry points', involved transferring cowpox material directly to the vaccinated person via a small ivory point.
4. Glycerinated lymph allowed the vaccinating material to be processed and preserved. It made possible large-scale sterile production.
5. R. N. Wilson, 'An Analysis of Fifty-Two cases of Tetanus Following Vaccine with Reference to the Source of Infection, 1839–1902', *Journal of the American Medical Association*, 38 (1902) pp. 1147, 1222; Joseph McFarland, 'Tetanus and Vaccination: An Analytical Study of 95 cases of the Complication', *Lancet* (1902) ii, 9, pp. 730–5; S. W. S. Toms, 'Tetanus Complicating Vaccine', *Medical News* (Philadelphia) 64 (1894) pp. 202–28.
6. Camden, New Jersey file, McFarland Papers, College of Physicians of Philadelphia.
7. Joseph McFarland, 'Report on the Camden Cases', see ibid.

8. Mulford had sold extensively in the Camden area and many pharmacists assumed that its product had been used. Letters file, McFarland Papers.

9. In December Mulford issued an advertisement defending glycerinated lymph. See Mulford Papers.

10. Camden file, McFarland Papers.

11. The other large Philadelphia area vaccine maker, H. M. Alexander, along with Mulford's main competitor, Parke Davis, both claimed to be doing good business in the Camden area.

12. Alexander did better business with state boards of health after the First World War, but at this time Mulford's claims were grander than Alexander's. See H. K. Mulford Company, 'Glycerinated Lymph', advertisements, 1900, Mulford Records; See also H. K. Mulford Company, 'The Exposure of a Disreputable Proceeding', copies in McFarland Papers and Mulford Records.

13. Interview, Dr J. H. Brown, 4 September 1980.

14. Mulford, 'Disreputable Proceeding'.

15. Ibid. *Pennsylvania State Board of Health, Annual Report* (1897) pp. 164–8, lists M. M. McKnight & Co. as owners.

16. US Hygienic Laboratory Records, National Archives, Public Health Service, General File (5016 Box 1) 'Report of the Division of Pathology and Bacteriology 1915', typescript, pp. 4–5.

17. Ibid.

18. *Pennsylvania Board, Annual Report* (1897) p. 167.

19. Mulford, 'Disreputable Proceedings'.

20. Ibid.

21. Ibid.

22. Ibid., pp. 11–12.

23. Ibid., p. 12. Mulford scarcely addressed, however, one problem which critics often raised, that the glycerine might affect the potency of the vaccine and have some possible link to tetanus. Both Walsh (in a letter to McFarland, 4 December 1901), and Alexander (letter to McFarland, 27 January 1902) shared this concern, but both had a strong stake in keeping this new technique. McFarland Papers.

24. Joseph McFarland, 'Vaccine Virus – Its Preparation and Complications Affecting its Use', *Journal of the American Medical Association*, 25 January 1902, p. 109.

25. H. M. Alexander to Joseph McFarland, 27 January 1902, in McFarland Papers.

26. H. M. Alexander to Joseph McFarland, 31 January 1902, in McFarland Papers.

27. 'Official Report of the Camden Board of Health Concerning Cases of Tetanus Which Occurred in Patients Who had been Vaccinated', in McFarlands Papers.

28. Ibid.

29. Ibid.

30. Whether or not the vaccine was contaminated in this case, vaccination was indeed somewhat risky because of the sores created. To combat this, vaccination shields were developed. Shortly after the 1901 outbreak, Mulford patented a shield which it tried to sell for regular use. Mulford's

non-patenting policy seems not to have extended to products other than drugs, though this was never made clear in their advertising, which claimed that the company allowed all their developments to be used for the general good. See shield in Division of Medical Sciences, Smithsonian Institution, and Mulford Catalogue, 1910, and patent, 1908.

31. 'Official Report of the Camden Board of Health'.
32. *Philadelphia Bureau of Health, Annual Report* (1902).
33. Ralph Walsh to McFarland, 4 December 1901, McFarland Papers.
34. Camden file, McFarland Papers.
35. Alexander to McFarland, 4 December 1901; Walsh to McFarland, 4 December and 14 December 1901.
36. Alexander to McFarland, 4 December 1901.
37. The National Vaccine Establishment had been founded in 1882 by Dr Ralph Walsh. Walsh had an MD from Georgetown University and during the Civil War was Acting Assistant Surgeon in the US Army Medical Corps. After the war he became a Professor of Physiology at Georgetown, until he opened his vaccine farm. The state of vaccines at the time, he claimed in his early advertising, was generally appalling.
38. Monkton Copeman, 'Glycerinated Vaccine', *Journal of Pathology and Bacteriology*, May 1891.
39. National Vaccine Establishment, 'The Laboratories of the National Vaccine Establishment, Washington', advertisement (n.d., circa 1901) in McFarland Papers. See also advertisements in Smithsonian Institution taken from the *American Public Health Journal*.
40. Alexander to McFarland, 20 January 1902, McFarland Papers.
41. Ibid.
42. Ibid.
43. Ibid.
44. Joseph McFarland, Paper presented to the Philadelphia County Medical Society, November 1901, in McFarland Papers.
45. Dr C. A. Hofer for H. K. Mulford and Company, letter to McFarland, 3 December 1901, in McFarland Papers. Hofer lost personal control over this sensitive issue after this first salvo at McFarland, and subsequent correspondence was carried on by his superiors, Henry Mulford and Milton Campbell.
46. Henry K. Mulford to McFarland, 6 December 1901, in McFarland Papers.
47. Smallpox statistics 1900–02 show the extent of the epidemic; see *Philadelphia Bureau of Health, Annual Reports*, 1900–02.
48. On New York see, Wayde Oliver, *The Man Who Lived for Tomorrow. William Hallock Park* (New York: Dutton, 1941); on Massachusetts see Barbara Rosenkrantz, *Public Health and the State, Conflict and Changing Views in Massachusetts 1842–1936* (Cambridge, Mass.: Harvard University Press, 1972) p. 123.
49. Rosenkrantz, *Public Health*, p. 123–4.
50. Advertisements in McFarland Papers.
51. Advertisements for Pocono Laboratory, n.d., 1901 and pamphlet of testimonials, in McFarland Papers.
52. Collected newspaper clippings, McFarland Papers.

53. Federal Act of 1 July 1902, 32 Stat L.; 728.
54. Ibid. The act was circulated as Department of Treasury Miscellaneous Publication No. 22 (1903).
55. United States Hygienic Laboratory Records, National Archives. Licence numbers had to be displayed on product labels and can be seen in the Smithsonian Institution, Division of Medical Sciences. See also Ramunas A. Kondratas, 'The US Hygienic Laboratory: Precursor to the National Institute of Health', unpublished typescript (Smithsonian Institution, 1980).
56. H. D. Geddings, Assistant Surgeon-General to Stein-Grey Drug Company, Cincinnati, Ohio, National Archives, Record Group 90, number 3655, box 340.
57. Note especially the career of J. J. Kinyoun, who moved from the directorship of the Hygienic Laboratory. He began work at H. K. Mulford in 1903, just as the act was being enforced. Milton Rosenau succeeded Kinyoun as Surgeon-General in 1899.
58. The Marine Hospital Service was one of the government's oldest agencies, founded in 1798 within the Department of the Treasury to provide for sick and infirm merchant marine sailors. See Lawrence F. Schmeckebier, *The Public Health Service, Its History, Activities and Organization* (Baltimore: Johns Hopkins University Press, 1923); A. Hunter Dupree, *Science in the Federal Government, A History of Policies and Activities to 1940* (Cambridge, Mass.: Harvard University Press, 1957) pp. 256–70; Ralph Chester Williams, *The United States Public Health Service 1798–1950* (Washington, DC: Commissioned Officers Association of the USPHS, 1950).
59. A. M. Stimson, 'A Brief History of Bacteriological Investigations of the United States Public Health Service', suppl. 141, *Public Health Reports* (Washington, DC: USGPO, 1938) p. 2. The purpose of this facility was to conduct routine tests on incoming ships and during the first year the presence of cholera was demonstrated among passengers on two vessels. Kinyoun made an effort to equip the laboratory with the best German apparatus and prided himself on possessing a microscope identical to that used by Koch, including the latest Zeiss lenses.
60. US Hygienic Laboratory Records, National Archives, 22 December 1908. This incident led to the closure of Mulford's Antitoxins from March 1909 to 30 December 1910. Mulford submitted a bill for $11 796.49 on 15 May 1909 for compensation which Wyman reluctantly paid.
61. Logbook for Hygienic Laboratory, 1902–04, Historical Collection, National Library of Medicine.
62. US Hygienic Laboratory Records, National Archives.
63. On Kinyoun and Rosenau see Williams, *Public Health Service*.
64. Ibid. United States Congress, Senate, *Hearings Before the Committee on Manufacturers . . . for preventing the Adulteration of Foods . . . Drugs . . .* 58th Congress, Report No. 1209 (Washington DC: USGPO, 1904) pp. 78–89, 96, 97.
65. Testimony of Mahlon H. Kline and Harvey Wiley, US Congress, *Hearings . . . Adulteration of Food*.
66. The 1906 Act can be seen as an extension of the law covering imports of

tea, approved 2 March 1883 and a law of 30 August 1890 covering food, drugs, and liquors.

67. Upton Sinclair, *The Jungle* (New York: Signet, 1960, first published 1905).

68. Large drug companies generally supported the passage of the 1906 Act, as can be seen from the Congressional Hearings.

69. Mahlon N. Kline, 'Some Reasons Why the Internal Revenue Tax on Alcohol Should be Reduced, and Why Our Government Should Provide Free Denaturized Alcohol for Use in the Arts', *American Journal of Pharmacy* (1905) p. 111.

70. US Congress, *Hearings . . . Adulteration of Foods*; M. N. Kline Tribute Book, SmithKline Archives.

71. M. N. Kline Tribute Book, SmithKline Archives.

72. 'Food and Drug Administration', SmithKline Archives.

73. United States Congress, 'An Act for Preventing the Manufacture, Sale, . . . of Adulterated Foods, Drugs, Medicines . . .', 34 Stat. 768 (1906).

74. J. Munch and J. Munch, Jr, 'The First Thousand Notices of Judgement under the Federal Food and Drug Legislation', *Food and Drug Journal* (1957) p. 219. Particularly significant sections of the act included section 4 which authorised chemical examinations, and section 7 which stated that a drug is adulterated if it 'differs from any official standard or falls below its own professed standards'. Numerous alterations to the act were incorporated until it was revised in 1938 by the Food, Drug and Cosmetics Act; see Peter Temin, *Taking Your Medicine. Drug Regulation in the United States* (Cambridge, Mass.: Harvard University Press) pp. 38–57.

75. Ibid., pp. 222–231.

76. In addition to its regulatory function, a great deal of pharmacological reasearch was undertaken in the drug laboratory. Kebler, supported by Wiley, wished to integrate research and regulatory activities. Thus elaborate facilities were established in 1909, complete with physiological testing apparatus, animal cages and surgical equipment. The character of the research followed other academic studies, for example of the effects of caffeine and the toxicity of alcohols. Wiley's successor in 1912, Carl L. Alsberg, divided the research and regulatory functions, shrinking the former while the latter grew inexorably. The research work had, in any case, been kept separate from the main concerns of the Bureau and with Alsberg it began to relate more closely to questions raised in the course of regulation. See *United States Public Health Service, Annual Report* (1909) pp. 437–8.

77. *United States Public Health Service, Annual Report* (1907) pp. 13–15. The hops and cod-liver oil studies were part of an even farther-reaching concern of the Agriculture Department, the export of domestic agricultural products. Hop growers had been preparing themselves for an export drive to sell the plant to British brewers when a scare was raised that their product was contaminated. The cod-liver oil studies were focused on the question of the supposed superiority of Norwegian oil over American.

78. Ibid.

79. *US Public Health Service, Annual Report* (1908) pp. 26–8.
80. The American Medical Association also lent its support to the passage of the 1906 Act as part of its anti-quackery activities.
81. *US Public Health Service, Annual Report* (1909) pp. 430.
82. Ibid., pp. 431.
83. Jonathan Liebenau, 'Dr Hand's Remedy: A Medical Vignette', *Pharmacy in History* (1987).
84. One of the clearest effects of the act was to reduce alcohol and narcotic content and to standardise state laws for those ingredients.
85. Hand's file, SmithKline Archive.
86. James Harvey Young, *Medical Messiahs* (Princeton: Princeton University Press, 1968) p. 44.
87. Ibid., pp. 3–12. See also Munch and Munch, 'Notices of Judgement', pp. 229–30.
88. Young, *Medical Messiahs*.
89. Munch and Munch, 'Notices of Judgement'.
90. Ibid.
91. Notices of Judgement 205 and 623, ibid.
92. Ibid.
93. Notice of Judgement 54, ibid.
94. Notice of Judgement 988, ibid., and p. 228.
95. Mahlon N. Kline, 'Digest of National Food and Drug Act and Regulations', pamphlet (Philadelphia: Smith Kline and French, 1907).
96. Willard Graham, *Pennsylvania Pharmaceutical Association, Proceedings*, (1908).
97. Ibid.
98. *US Public Health Service, Annual Report* (1916).
99. Testimony of Mahlon Kline, US Congress, *Hearings . . . Adulteration of Foods*.
100. *US Public Health Service, Annual Report* (1917) p. 13, Alsberg report.
101. Ibid., p. 14.
102. Ibid.
103. Hygienic Laboratory Records, National Archives.
104. US Congress, *Hearings . . . Adulteration of Foods*.
105. Ibid.
106. Young, *Medical Messiahs*.
107. Dupree, *Science in the Federal Government*, pp. 268–9; Temin, *Taking Your Medicine*, p. 27ff.

CHAPTER 7

1. Alfred D. Chandler, *The Visible Hand. The Managerial Revolution in American Business* (Cambridge, Mass.: Harvard University Press, 1977) p. 375.
2. James Harvey Young, *The Medical Messiahs: A Social History of Health Quackery in Twentieth-Century America* (Princeton: Princeton University Press, 1967) pp. 60–2.
3. John Thomas Mahoney, *The Merchants of Life. An Account of the*

American Pharmaceutical Industry (New York: Harper, 1959) pp. 156–81.

4. Ibid., p. 162.
5. Ibid., p. 163.
6. United States Laboratory Records, National Archives.
7. Mahoney, *Merchants*, p. 163.
8. Ibid.
9. Ibid., p. 198. This was only one-fifteenth of their needs, but was important because of the political capital the department was able to make of it due to their continuing inability to convince the city government that they needed more money to establish a larger antitoxin laboratory themselves. See *Philadelphia Bureau of Health, Annual Reports* (1896–1910).
10. 'Elixir Viburnum and Hydrastis Compound (Uterine Sedative)', pamphlet No. 138 (1897) Wyeth Records.
11. 'Remarks on Fermentative Dyspepsia', pamphlet No. 67 (1894) Wyeth Records.
12. 'Chromium Sulphate', pamphlet No. 100 (1908); 'Hypodermic Tablets Containing Mercury Succinimide', pamphlet No. 101 (1909); 'Glycoesophates', pamphlet No. 102. (1905); 'Plastules'. pamphlet No. 107 (1913) and others; see book of pamphlets, Wyeth Records.
13. Wyeth Ledger, Wyeth Records.
14. 'Analytical Laboratory Notes', 1908, SmithKline Records.
15. Ibid. C. Mahlon Kline was groomed for the leadership of the company since he attended the William Penn Charter School.
16. England was a prominent person already at the Philadelphia Hospital, 'where, under his direction, over 1 583 000 prescriptions were safely compounded, and where he was very closely associated with many prominent physicians, and was editor of the Philadelphia Hospital Formulary', ibid., p. 39.
17. Smith Kline Ledger, 1898–1902, SmithKline Archive.
18. 'Smith Kline and French', *Pharmaceutical Era*, 31 December 1896, p. 957.
19. See Rima B. Apple, '"To Be Used Only Under the Direction of A Physician": Commercial Infant Feeding and Medical Practice, 1870–1940', *Bulletin of the History of Medicine*, 54 (1980) pp. 402–17.
20. Harry B. French to J. W. England, 12 January 1901, in SmithKline Records.
21. Ibid.
22. H. B. French to J. W. England, 4 February 1916, in SmithKline Records.
23. J. G. Roberts to William Eiman, 12 March 1953, in SmithKline Records.
24. Ibid.
25. 'Analytical Laboratory Notes', 1907, SmithKline Records.
26. Smith Kline and French, *Annual Report*, 1908, p. 41.
27. Roberts to Eiman.
28. Photo file, SmithKline Archive.
29. Smith Kline advertisement, *Pharmaceutical Record*, 1891, p. 10. See also advertisement file in SmithKline Records. The company expanded continuously until Sharp and Dohme moved to Philadelphia and disrupted the balance of the local drug trade. The company suffered its second major retreat since the Civil War, cutting production, laying off workers and

sparking labour unrest which was not resolved until the company agreed to retain all workers on a two-day basis. See Tom Fehnenberger, file, SmithKline Archive.

30. 'Analytical Report', 1908, p. 3, SmithKline Records.

31. J. Roberts, *Digest of Researches by Laboratory Workers of the Smith, Kline and French Company*, vol I, comprising abstracts of papers published from 1893–1904, SmithKline Records.

32. Willard Graham, 'Laboratory Notes', *American Journal of Pharmacy* (1904) p. 389.

33. C. M. Kline, 'African Balsam of Copaiba', *American Journal of Pharmacy* (1904) p. 176 and (1905) p. 185.

34. Joseph England, 'Tincture of Nux Vomica, 1900', *American Journal of Pharmacy* (1906) p. 527.

35. George Pancoast and Willard Graham, 'Commercial Volatile Oils of the Coniferae', *Pennsylvania Pharmaceutical Association, Proceedings*, (1905).

36. Pearson's publication record was probably an aid when he applied for the professorship of chemistry.

37. See, for example, W. Pearson, 'The Pharmacopoeia from the Viewpoint of an Analytical Worker', *American Journal of Pharmacy* (1907) p. 75; and *American Druggist*, 10 February 1908.

38. W. Pearson, 'Standardization of Diphtheria Antitoxin', *Pennsylvania Pharmaceutical Association, Proceedings* (1907).

39. Pearson was encouraged to continue his work on antitoxin despite the fact that Smith Kline did not deal in the product. The tone of the article, furthermore, was helpful. It explained to pharmacists why they should keep the serum under proper conditions by educating them about the characteristics and standards of commercial preparations.

40. Mahlon Kline, 'Congressional Testimony, 1906', Transcript in Smith-Kline Records.

41. 'Historical Fragment: A Century of Service', 1945?, unpublished manuscript in SmithKline Records.

42. Arnold Thackray, Robert Bud, P. Thomas Carroll and Jeffrey Sturchio, *Chemistry in America, 1876–1976: Historical Indicators* (Dordrecht: Reidel, 1985).

43. One of the first tasks after the 1906 Act was passed was to reformulate medicines such as Hand's Cholic Cure which would otherwise violate some aspects of the law. Hypnotics and opiates were generally removed or at least reduced and replaced by comparable but seemingly less harmful drugs, while old remedies were analysed and their contents specified. The law had made other requirements too: scientists were necessary to ensure that standards were maintained and even to interpret the criteria for complete labelling. Aside from the bacteriologically trained 'responsible head' required by the 1902 Act for producers of biologicals, it was understood that a large staff of bacteriologists and physiologists should be on hand to test the purity and quality of serums, vaccines and toxins.

CHAPTER 8

1. See for example, the H. K. Mulford Company's Code of Ethics, Mulford Records, Merck and Company, West Point, Pennsylvania.

2. Jonathan Liebenau, 'The Use of American Patents by German and American Industries, 1890–1935', unpublished typescript, University of Pennsylvania, 1978. In 1902 the number of patents taken out in the United States by Germans surpassed the number assigned to Britons. Chemical manufacturers accounted for a large number of these. See Williams Haynes, *American Chemical Industry: A History*, Vol. 3 (New York: van Nostrand, 1945–52) p. 481. See also *US Patent Commission, Annual Reports 1890–1935* (Washington, DC: US Patent Office).

3. F. A. Seely, 'International Protection of Industrial Property', *Proceedings and Addresses, Celebration of the Beginning of the Second Century of the American Patent System at Washington City, D. C., April 8, 1891* (Washington, DC: Gedney and Roberts, 1892) pp. 199–216. See also G. F. Folk, *Patents and Industrial Progress* (New York: Harper, 1942).

4. The procedure for obtaining a United States patent had become routinised in at least two German chemical firms. By 1905 Hoechst and BASF had offset forms for their chemists to fill out in order to apply for an American patent. These forms automatically assigned the patent to the company and specified American legal agents. See patent records in the Center for Polar and Scientific Archives, National Archives, Washington, DC.

5. For the use of patents to 'patent around' in the electronics industry, see Leonard S. Reich, 'Radio Electronics and the Development of Industrial Research in the Bell System', PhD dissertation, Johns Hopkins University, 1977, pp. 171–4. Reich believes that companies used patents 'both offensively and defensively: either to gain concessions from competitors, or to short-circuit new inventions which might have had disruptive possibilities. In almost every case, research became an important facet of competition for monopoly control rather than competition for shares of the market' (p. 174). See also David F. Nobel, *America by Design: Science, Technology and the Rise of Corporate Capitalism* (New York: Knopf, 1977) pp. 95–110.

6. Haynes, *Chemical Industry*, Vol. 3, pp. 311–15.

7. Advertisement, *Journal of the American Medical Association*, 13 January 1917, p. 47.

8. US Patent Office, *Patent Lists*, 1898–1912.

9. The patents in question were: No. 1 081 592 ('Salvarsan', granted 16 December 1913) to Paul Ehrlich and Alfred Bertheim, assignors to Farbwerke vorm, Meister Lucius u. Bruning (Hoechst); No. 1 081 897 (16 December 1913); and No. 1 116 398 (10 November 1914). See Patent Records, National Archives. These, and other key Hoechst products were signed over to Metz under a standing agreement which was explained in congressional testimony 23 March 1922, see US Congress, Senate, *Hearings Before the Subcommittee of the Judiciary on the Alleged Dye Monopoly*, 67th Congress, 1st Session, 1922, Testimony of Mr Herman A. Metz (Washington, DC: USGPO) pp. 741–55. See also Paul

Ehrlich and S. Hata, *Die Experimentelle Chemotherapie der Spirilossen* (Berlin: Springer, 1910).

10. On Metz see *Who Was Who in America*, Vol. 1, p. 835; *National Cyclopedia of American Biography*, Vol. 14, pp. 347–8. A flamboyant and highly successful businessman and politician, Metz is an excellent candidate for a biography.
11. US Congress, *Alleged Dye Monopoly*, p. 742.
12. Ibid., p. 749.
13. Ibid., p. 753.
14. Ibid., p. 749.
15. Ibid.
16. The U-boat *Deutschland* was a cargo-carrying submarine used to avoid the British blockade. She made two trips for Metz in July and November 1916 carrying around one million dollars-worth of cargo each time. Ibid., p. 812.
17. Patricia Spain Ward, 'The American Reception of Salvarsan', *Journal of the History of Medicine and Allied Science*, 35 (1980).
18. Ibid.; John B. Murphy, 'The Arsenical Treatment of Syphilis', *Journal of the American Medical Association*, 55 (1910) pp. 1113–15; Abraham L. Wolbarst, 'Ehrlich's Arsenobenzol: Its Technique and Indications for General Use', *New York Medical Journal*, 92 (1910) pp. 972–4.
19. Maria Marquardt, *Paul Ehrlich* (London: 1949); Claude E. Dolman, 'Paul Ehrlich', *Dictionary of Scientific Biography*, Vol. 4 (New York: Scribner, 1974) pp. 295–305.
20. Ward, 'Reception of Salvarsan'.
21. The papers of the Dermatological Research Laboratories are in the College of Physicians of Philadelphia. Hereafter they will be referred to as DRL Papers. On the DRL see John A. Kolmer, 'History of the Research Institute of Cutaneous Medicine', in Ruben Friedman (ed.) *A History of Dermatology in Philadelphia* (Fort Pierce Beach, Florida: Froben, 1955) pp. 307–15; Aaron Litchin and Ira Leo Schamberg, 'The Dawn of American-Made Synthetic Drugs', unpublished manuscript, copy in Kremers Reference Files, University of Wisconsin School of Pharmacy Library; Dermatological Research Laboratory, 'Abstract of Minutes of the First Meeting . . . March 3rd, 1921', in DRL Papers.
22. On the founder, Schamberg, see F. D. Weidman, 'Memoir of Jay Frank Schamberg, M.D.', *College of Physicians of Philadelphia Transactions*, 2, series 4 (1934) pp. xii–xiv; Ira Leo Schamberg, 'A. C. Barnes, M.D., vs. J. F. Schamberg, M.D.: A Chemotherapeutic Confrontation', *Transactions and Studies of the College of Physicians of Philadelphia*, 41, series 4 (1974) pp. 289–94. Obituaries of Schamberg were printed in the *Archives of Dermatology and Syphilology*, 29 (1934) pp. 901–4; *Journal of the American Medical Association*, 102 (1934) p. 1245; the *Pennsylvanian Medical Journal*, 37 (1934) pp. 671–3; and *Dermatologische Wochenschrift*, (1934) pp. 1114–15. See also Louis Pelner, 'Jay Frank Schamberg, M.D. (1870–1934), Medical Scholar and Founder of the Independent American Pharmaceutical Industry', *Medical Times*, 97, No. 12 (1969) pp. 95–1000; A. Lichtin and Ira Leo Schamberg, 'Jay Frank Schamberg, A Pioneer in Dermatologic Research and

Chemotherapy', *AMA Archives of Dermatology*, 73 (1956) p. 493; Sigmund S. Greenbaum, and Carroll S. Wright, 'Memoir of J. Frank Schamberg, M.D. (1870–1934)', *Urologic and Cutaneous Review*, 51 (1947) pp. 251–3. On Kolmer see his vita and miscellaneous material in the Papers of John Allert Kolmer, College of Physicians of Philadelphia; 'Memoir of John A. Kolmer', *College of Physicians of Philadelphia, Transactions*, 32, series 4 (1965) p. 49. Also his own 'History of the Research Institute'.

23. I. L. Schamberg, 'A. C. Barnes'; Weidman, 'Memoir'. This is apparent from his style of correspondence in the DRL Papers.

24. DRL, *Publications from the D.R.L. of Philadelphia, Collected Reprints*, 2 vols. Copy in the Library of Congress, 1918, 1920; 'List of Articles Published from the Dermatological Research Laboratories', DRL Papers. The first work of the staff was to produce treatments for skin disorders: 'In the course of early investigations the staff produced a number of new medicinal chemical compounds, chiefly mercurial compounds, one of which, known as mercurophen, came into wide use as one of the most valuable antiseptics known to medical science'. Kolmer, 'History of the Research Institute', p. 307.

25. Kolmer was a fantastically productive scientist, publishing over twenty papers in some years, usually in collaboration with his laboratory assistants. Raiziss published primarily new syntheses, leaving it to his associates to test and apply them.

26. Although they held full academic appointments at the University of Pennsylvania, they had little access to laboratory facilities there.

27. George Washington Corner, *Two Centuries of Medicine. A History of the School of Medicine, University of Pennsylvania* (Philadelphia: Lippincott, 1965) pp. 215*ff*. The DRL, on the other hand, was very well funded. Salaries were based on the level given at the Rockefeller Institute, and Raiziss earned $15 000 a year, Kolmer and Schamberg $12 000 each. US Congress, *Alleged Dye Monopoly*, p. 917.

28. 'Widener', DRL Papers; US Congress, *Alleged Dye Monopoly*, p. 917.

29. Ibid.; I. L. Schamberg, 'A. C. Barnes'; 'P. A. B. Widener', *Dictionary of American Biography* (New York: Scribners, 1929–46).

30. E. Digby Baltzell, *An American Business Aristocracy* (New York: Collier, 1962) pp. 147–8, 190.

31. J. F. Schamberg, J. A. Kolmer, A. I. Ringer and G. W. Raiziss, 'Research Studies in Psoriasis', *Journal of Cutaneous Diseases*, 31 (1913) pp. 698, 803.

32. J. A. Kolmer and J. F. Schamberg, 'The Clinical Interpretation of the Wasserman Reaction with Special Reference to Cholesterinized Antigens', *College of Physicians of Philadelphia, Transactions*, October 1914; J. F. Schamberg, J. A. Kolmer and G. W. Raiziss, 'A Study of the Germicidal Activity of Chrysarobin and Certain other Medicaments Used in Psoriasis', *Journal of Cutaneous Diseases*, 32 (1914) p. 85.

33. J. F. Schamberg, A. I. Ringer, G. W. Raiziss, J. A. Kolmer, 'Summary of Research Studies in Psoriasis', *Journal of the American Medical Association*, 63 (1914) p. 729. Oliver S. Ormsby and James Herbert Mitchell (eds) *Skin and Venereal Diseases (Yearbook of Dermatology*

and Syphilology) (Chicago: Year Book Publishers, 1915).
34. Correspondence file, 1914, DRL Papers.
35. Kolmer, 'History of the Research Institute'; see advertisement in *Progress of Chemotherapy and the Treatment of Syphilis*, 1 (1924).
36. US Congress, *Alleged Dye Monopoly*, pp. 982, 1006; 'D.R.L. Correspondence – and papers concerning the German Farbwerke drug patents, 1914–1922', DRL Papers; Ormsby and Mitchell, *Skin and Venereal Diseases (Yearbook of Dermatology and Syphilology)* (Chicago: Yearbook Publishers, 1916) p. 222.
37. US Patents Nos. 937 929; 1 081 592; 1 081 897; 1 116 398. Copies in Record Group 241, National Archives. Kolmer, 'History of the Research Institute'; J. Schumacher, 'Das Salvarsen, ein echter Farbstoff', *Dermatologische Wochenschrift*, 47 (1914) pp. 1295–304.
38. Ibid., Ward, 'American Reception'.
39. George B. Roth, 'An Experimental Investigation of the Toxicity of Certain Organic Arsenic Compounds', *US Hygienic Laboratory Bulletins*, No. 113 (Washington, DC: USGPO, 1918). Aside from 'Salvarsan', manufactured by Hoechst (and H. A. Metz Laboratories after the war). 'Kharsivan' was produced by Wellcome Laboratories in Britain. 'Arsenobillion' by Billion Freres in France, 'Diarsenol' by the Synthetic Drug Company in Canada, and 'Arsaminol' in Japan. The official American name, 'Arsenobenzol', was later used by Squibb and Powers, Weightman and Rosengarten (which was acquired by Merck and Company in 1927) in addition to the DRL.
40. American patent law allows for the production but not the sale of products covered by unexpired patents. The DRL was not infringing on Metz's production rights as long as they used the medicine for experimental purposes.
41. 'Correspondence', DRL Papers.
42. US Congress, *Alleged Dye Monopoly*, p. 869.
43. J. F. Schamberg, paper presented to the Medical Society of the State of Pennsylvania, 22 September 1915, in DRL Papers. See also the subsequent resolution, letter C. L. Stevens, 6 October 1915.
44. 'Correspondence', DRL Papers.
45. John H. Stokes to Franklin H. Martin, 13 March 1917, DRL Papers.
46. Ibid., US Congress, *Alleged Dye Monopoly*, pp. 980, 994–6; Herman A. Metz to 'The Medical Profession', March 1917, DRL Papers.
47. Diary of phone conversations, meetings, etc., 6 November 1916 to 1 June 1917, DRL Papers.
48. United States Congress, Senate, *Hearings Before the Committee of Patents on Salvarsan*, 65th Congress, 1st session, 1917, pp. 8–9; Stokes to Martin, 13 March 1917, DRL Papers.
49. Stokes to Martin, 13 March 1917.
50. US Congress, *Alleged Dye Monopoly*, pp. 985–6; copies of the agreement are in the DRL Papers.
51. Jay F. Schamberg, J. A. Kolmer, and G. W. Raiziss, 'The Administration of Arsenobenzol by Mouth', *Journal of the American Medical Association*, 67 (1916) p. 1919; *United States Pharmacopoeia* (Philadelphia: 1920).

52. United States Congress, *Alleged Dye Monopoly*, pp. 987*ff*; Metz to 'The Medical profession', March 1917.
53. 'List of Articles Published From Dermatological Research Laboratories', DRL Papers.
54. 'Correspondence', 'Advertisements', DRL Papers.
55. Roth, 'Toxicity'; George B. Roth, 'The Biological Standardisation of Arsephenamine and Neoarsphenamine', *US Hygienic Laboratory Bulletins*, No. 135 (Washington DC: USGPO, 1923); Jay F. Schamberg, John A. Kolmer and Geroge W. Raiziss, 'Comparative Studies of the Toxicity of Arsphenamine and Neoarsphenamine', *American Journal of Medical Science*, 140 (1920) p. 188. See also H. Sheridan Baketel, 'On the Use of American Made Salvarsan', *American Journal of Syphilology*, 2 (1918) p. 544–9. Baketel worked for Herman Metz and promoted this product over the DRL Arsenobenzol on grounds of quality, lower toxicity and ease of use.
56. US Congress, *Alleged Dye Monopoly*, p. 869; 'Correspondence', DRL Papers.
57. Ibid.
58. Stokes to Martin, 13 March 1917.
59. US Congress, *Salvarsan*, referring to S. 2178.
60. Ibid., referring to S. 2363.
61. Ibid.
62. Ibid., p. 8–15.
63. Editor, 'Abrogate the Patent on Salvarsan', *Journal of the American Medical Association*, 68 (1917) p. 1187.
64. Metz to 'The Medical Profession', March 1917.
65. Ibid.
66. Ibid.
67. Hearings were held on various aspects of the patent controversy in reference to the German dye companies.
68. United States Congress, 'Trading with the Enemy Act' ('Adamson Bill') 40 stat. h., 420, approved 12 October 1917.
69. DRL licence, DRL Papers.
70. US Congress, *Alleged Dye Monopoly*, p. 996; 'Correspondence', DRL Papers.
71. *New and Non-Official Remedies* (Washington DC: 1916); Haynes, *American Chemical Industry*, Vol. 3, pp. 318–20.
72. Ibid.
73. US Congress, *Alleged Dye Monopoly*, pp. 982–3, 991. Correspondence with the Philadelphia Polyclinic College for Graduates in Medicine, DRL Papers.
74. Compare, for example, the claims made by the DRL with Mulford's claims for antimeningitis serum.
75. *Mulford Digest*, 1 (1900), see Chapter 5. The similarity goes a little further than that, since in 1917 the DRL contracted Mulford to supply foreign markets.
76. *Progress of Chemotherapy and the Treatment of Syphilis.*
77. US Congress, *Alleged Dye Monopoly*, p. 872.
78. Ibid., p. 1001.

79. Ibid., p. 918.
80. Ibid., pp. 873–4.
81. 'Gustav Metz', in Williams Haynes, *Who's Who in Chemical Industry* (New York: 1928).
82. 'H. Sheridan Baketel', in ibid.; also Baketel, 'American Made Salvarsan'.
83. Ibid.
84. US Congress, *Alleged Dye Monopoly*, p. 872, and Metz Advertisements, DRL Papers.
85. Ibid.
86. Haynes, *Chemical Industry*, Vol. 3 pp. 281. 284*ff*, 292; DRL 'Abstract of Minutes,' DRL Papers.
87. Ibid., US Congress, *Alleged Dye Monopoly*, pp. 1001, 1004.
88. The net profit of the DRL amounted to nearly $¾ million by 1919. Ibid.; 'Correspondence with Abbott Laboratories', DRL Papers.
89. Ibid., 'Dermatological Research Institute', DRL Papers.
90. 'Schamberg', DRL Papers.
91. Ibid.
92. 'Correspondence with Abbott Laboratories', DRL Papers. Ties with Abbott had begun in 1917, see Alfred S. Burdick to Jay Frank Schamberg, 21 June 1917, DRL Papers.
93. Herman Kogan, *The Long White Line. The Story of Abbott Laboratories* (New York: Random House, 1963) p. 111.
94. Ibid., pp. 110–13; 'Correspondence with Abbott', DRL Papers.
95. Kogan, *Abbott Laboratories*, pp. 111–13.
96. Ibid.
97. Ibid., p. 112.
98. Ibid., p. 113–14; 'Correspondence with Abbott', 16 October 1922, 18 October 1922, 19 October 1922, DRL Papers; John Thomas Mahoney, *The Merchants of Life. An Account of the American Pharmaceutical Industry* (New York: Harper, 1959) pp. 136–8.
99. Kogan, *Abbott Laboratories*, pp. 110–13.
100. Ibid., File, 1922–23, DRL Papers.
101. Ibid., 'Raymond E. Horn', *Who's Who in Chemical Industry*.
102. Kogan, *Abbott Laboratories*.
103. 'Correspondence with Abbott', DRL Papers.
104. Ibid.

CHAPTER 9

1. As was the case at Smith Kline where a distinct aspect of Lyman Kebler's laboratory was to reproduce products made by Parke Davis, Mulford and others.
2. The trade catalogues of competing companies from 1900–20 appear remarkably similar both in range of products and price. Differences in quality were similarly reduced by competition.
3. For example, Mulford and others marketed combinations of quinine with

arsenous acid, iron and strychnine. See H. K. Mulford Company, *Price List* (1900) p. 545.

4. William D. Rubenstein, *Men of Property* (London: Croom Helm, 1981) pp. 247–8.

5. Informal knowledge is in many cases crucial to reproducing scientific results. See, for example Elting Morrison, *From Nowhere to Know How* (Cambridge, Mass.: MIT Press, 1976); Patricia Woole, 'The Second Messinger: Informal Communication in Cyclic AMP Research', *Minerva*, 14 (1976) pp. 349–73; H. M. Collins, 'The TEA Set: Tacit Knowledge and Scientific Networks', *Science Studies*, 4 (1974) pp. 164–86.

6. The strength of the industry after the war can be seen by the total value of druggists' preparations and chemicals mainly distributed through the drug trade, which in 1923 was $425 102 073. Most of this was non-proprietary tinctures, extracts and syrups, while biological products accounted for $13 892 495. C. H. Waterbury (for the Committee on Proprietary Goods), *How to Get it – Also Decisions Governing Distribution. A Manual for Manufacturers, Proprietors, Advertisers, Advertising Agencies and Buyers – Practical Answers to Practical Problems* (New York: National Wholesale Druggists' Association, 1923) p. 59. See also Williams Haynes, *The American Chemical Industry: A History*, Vol. 3 (New York: Van Nostrand, 1950) pp. 245*ff*.

7. For Mulford see Chapter 5; for the DRL see Chapter 8.

8. The stigma associated with patenting medicines and devices seems to have been removed during the 1920s and most companies took out patents on their important products, often advertising the fact in catalogues.

9. See US Hygienic Laboratory Records, National Archives.

10. See Chapter 8.

11. Herman Kogan, *The Long White Line. The Story of Abbott Laboratories* (New York: Random House, 1963) pp. 91*ff*; John Thomas Mahoney, *The Merchants of Life. An Account of the American Pharmaceutical Industry* (New York: Harper, 1959) p. 137.

12. James G. Burrow, *AMA: Voice of American Medicine* (Baltimore: Johns Hopkins University Press, 1963) pp. 16–26.

13. John Parascandola, 'Industrial Research Comes of Age: The American Pharmaceutical Industry, 1920–1940', *Pharmacy in History*, 27 (1985) pp. 12–21 and 'John J. Abel and the Founding of ASPET', *The Pharmacologist*, 26 (1984) pp. 37–40.

14. Ibid., see also Mahoney, *Merchants of Life*, p. 8.

15. Abraham Flexner, *Medical Education in the United States and Canada* (New York: Carnegie Foundation, 1910); Gerald E. Markowitz and David Rosner, 'Doctors in Crisis: Medical Education and Medical Reform During the Progressive Era, 1895–1915', in Susan Reverby and David Rosner (eds) *Health Care in America, Essays in Social History* (Philadelphia: Temple University Press, 1979) pp. 184–205.

16. David L. Cowen, 'Materia Medica and Pharmacology' in Ronald L. Numbers (ed.) *The Education of American Physicians: Historical Essays* (Berkeley: University of California Press, 1980) pp. 95–121; and John Parascandola, 'John J. Abel and the Early Development of Pharmacology at Johns Hopkins University', *Bulletin of the History of Medicine*, 56

(1982) pp. 512–27. See also the excellent work by John Patrick Swann, 'The Emergence of Cooperative Research Between American Universities and the Pharmaceutical Industry, 1920–1940', PhD dissertation, University of Wisconsin, Madison, 1985.

17. Ibid.
18. See Parascandola, 'Industrial Research'.
19. Flexner, *Medical Education*.
20. George Washington Corner, *Two Centuries of Medicine. A History of the School of Medicine, University of Pennsylvania* (Philadelphia: Lippincott, 1965) pp. 229–33.
21. Physicians were full-time members of the research staffs at Mulford, Parke Davis and elsewhere.
22. Peter Steckl, 'Biological Standardization of Drugs Before 1928', PhD dissertation, University of Wisconsin, 1969; M. K. Weikel, 'Research as a Function of the Pharmaceutical Industry, the American Formative Period', MA thesis, University of Wisconsin, 1962.
23. Ibid.
24. Ibid.
25. Birdsey L. Maltbie, *A Quarter Century of Progress in Manufacturing Pharmacy* (New York: American Pharmaceutical Manufacturers' Association, 1937).
26. Smith Kline Catalogues, 1900–20, SmithKline Papers.
27. Sharpe and Dohme Catalogues, 1900–20, Merck Papers.
28. Parke Davis Catalogues, 1900–20, Smithsonian Institution; Mulford Catalogues, Mulford Papers.
29. Parke Davis, Advertisements, *Philadelphia College of Pharmacy, Alumni Reports*, 1895–1905.
30. Mahlon Kline Correspondence, SmithKline Papers.
31. 'Eskay' file, SmithKline Papers.
32. Ibid.; Joseph England file, SmithKline Papers.
33. Ibid., Rima D. Apple, '"To Be Used Only Under the Direction of a Physician": Commercial Infant Feeding and Medical Practice, 1870–1940', *Bulletin of the History of Medicine*, 54 (1980) pp. 402–17.
34. Ibid.
35. Analytical Laboratory file, SmithKline Papers.
36. Mulford and Sharp and Dohme Merger file, Mulford Papers; see also Chapter 8.
37. Ibid.
38. Ibid.
39. Ibid.
40. Plant Descriptions, Mulford Papers.
41. Sharp and Dohme papers, Merck Archive. The poor state of their research is evident from catalogues, which show virtually no innovative products.
42. Ibid.
43. Ibid.
44. Ibid.
45. Glenolden File, Mulford Papers.
46. Phillip Richard Hackett, 'Consolidation in the Drug Industry', PhD

dissertation, University of Illinois (Urbana), 1932.

47. Ibid.

48. W. H. Helfand, H. B. Woodruff, K. M. H. Coleman, D. L. Cowen, 'Wartime Industrial Development of Penicillin in the United States', in John Parascandola (ed.) *The History of Antibiotics: A Symposium* (Madison: American Institute of the History of Pharmacy, 1980) pp. 31–56.

49. Selman A. Waksman, *My Life with the Microbes* (New York: Simon and Schuster, 1954) pp. 245–55.

50. D. Schwartzman, *Innovation in the Pharmaceutical Industry* (Baltimore: Johns Hopkins University Press, 1976).

51. United States Congress, Senate, *Hearing Before the Subcommittee on Antitrust and Monopoly of the Committee of the Judiciary on Administered Prices*, 86th Congress, 2nd session, 1959.

Bibliography

MANUSCRIPT COLLECTIONS

Company repositories

American Home Products, Narberth, Pennsylvania:
   Wyeth Laboratories Papers
Merck and Company, West Point, Pennsylvania:
   H. K. Mulford Papers
   Powers and Weightman Papers
   Rosengarten and Son Papers
   Sharp and Dohme Papers
SmithKline Corporation, Philadelphia, Pennsylvania:
   Dr Hand's Remedies Papers
   Smith Kline and French Papers
   SKF Products Division
Arthur H. Thomas Company, Philadelphia, Pennsylvania:
   Arthur H. Thomas Papers

Other repositories

Dr John H. Brown, Marietta, Pennsylvania:
   H. M. Alexander Company Papers
College of Physicians of Philadelphia, Pennsylvania:
   Dermatological Research Laboratories Papers
   John Albert Kolmer Papers
   Joseph McFarland Papers
   H. M. Metz Laboratories Papers
   William Swaim Papers
   Trade Catalogue Collection
Elutherian Mills-Hagley Foundation, Wilmington, Delaware:
   Troth Company Papers
Historical Society of Pennsylvania, Philadelphia:
   Philadelphia Drug Exchange Papers
National Archives, Washington, DC:
   Hygienic Laboratory Records
   Patent Office Records
Philadelphia City Archives, Pennsylvania:
   Public Health Department Papers

Smithsonian Institution, Washington, DC:
  Aimer Pharmacy Papers
  Division of Medical Sciences Trade Catalogue Collection
  Warshaw Collection
University of Pennsylvania Archive, Philadelphia:
  Laboratory of Hygiene Papers

UNITED STATES PATENTS

Alexander, H. M., No. 710 234, 'Vaccine Container', 20 September 1902.

Behring, Emil (assigned to Hoechst), No. 606 042, 'Diphtheria Antitoxin', 21 June 1898.

Ehrlich, Paul with A. Bertheim (assigned to Hoechst), No. 909 380, 'Arsenophenol', 12 January 1909; No. 937 929, 'Derivative of Aminoarylarsinic Acid', 26 October 1909; No. 986 148, 'Salvarsan', 7 March 1911; No. 986 544, 'Salvarsan', 7 March 1911; No. 1 078 135, 'Neo-salvarsan', 11 November 1913; No. 1 081 592, 'Neo-salvarsan', 16 December 1913.

Gill, John F. (assigned to Henry Bower, Wyeth Brothers), No. 215 452, 'Tablet Machine', 28 March 1879.

Lusby, John (assigned to Wyeth Brothers), No. 323 349, 'Tablet Machine', 1885.

Morris, Abraham R. (assigned to H. K. Mulford), No. 617 255, 'Tablet Machine', 3 January 1899.

Smith, Oberlin and Henry K. Mulford, No. 413 310, 'Machine for Manufacturing Compressed Pills', 22 October 1889.

Walsh, Ralph, No. 742 762, 'Glycerinated Vaccine Syringe', 23 October 1903; Nos 766 203 and 766 204, 'Syringes', 2 August 1904.

UNPUBLISHED SOURCES

Becker, William, 'Wholesalers of Hardware and Drugs, 1870–1900', PhD dissertation, Johns Hopkins University, 1969.

Blancher, David, 'Workshops of the Bacteriological Revolution: A History of the Laboratories of the New York City Department of Health, 1892–1912', PhD dissertation, City University of New York, 1979.

Eisenberg, Albert C., 'A General Survey of Production and Wages in Twenty-One Philadelphia Industries, 1925–1931', MBA thesis, University of Pennsylvania, 1935.

Garipy, Thomas, 'The Reception of Listerism in America', MA thesis, Notre Dame University, 1976.

Hackett, Robert Phillip, 'Consolidation in the Drug Industry', MA thesis, University of Illinois (Urbana), 1932.

Hook, George B., 'An Historical Evaluation of the American Drug Market Since 1900', PhD dissertation, University of Pittsburgh, 1955.

Kondratas, Ramunas A., 'The U.S. Hygienic Laboratory: Precursor to the National Institute of Health', typescript, Smithsonian Institution, 1980.

Liebenau, Jonathan, 'German-Held American Patents, 1890–1930', type-script, University of Pennsylvania, 1978.

Liebenau, Jonathan, 'The Reception of Antisepsis in the United States', paper presented to the American Association for the History of Medicine, 1978.

Liebenau, Jonathan, 'Medicine and Technology', paper presented to the British Society for the History of Science, 1980.

McEvilla, Joseph D., 'Competition in the American Pharmaceutical Industry', PhD dissertation, University of Pittsburgh, 1955.

McFadyen, Richard E., 'Estes Kefauver and the Drug Industry', PhD dissertation, Emory University, 1973.

O'Hara, Leo J., 'An Emerging Profession, Philadelphia Medicine, 1860–1900', PhD dissertation, University of Pennsylvania, 1976.

Parascandola, John, 'The Rise of Pharmacology in the United States', typescript, University of Wisconsin, 1979.

Reich, Leonard S., 'Radio Electronics and the Development of Industrial Research in the Bell System', PhD dissertation, Johns Hopkins University, 1977.

Steckl, Peter, 'Biological Standardization of Drugs Before 1928', PhD dissertation, University of Wisconsin, 1969.

Weikel, Malcolm Keith, 'Research as a Function of the Pharmaceutical Industry, The American Formative Period', MA thesis, University of Wisconsin, 1962.

Yaeger, Mary, 'Beyond "The Jungle": The Changing Economics and Politics of Food Control', paper presented to the Smithsonian Institution, 1979.

CONGRESSIONAL HEARINGS

United States Congress, Senate, *Hearings Before the Committee on Manufacturers . . . For Preventing the Adulteration of Foods . . . Drugs*, 58th Congress, 2nd session, 1904.

United States Congress, Senate, *Hearings Before the Committee on Patents on Salvarsan*, 65th Congress 1st session, 1917.

United States Congress, Senate, *Hearings Before the Subcommittee of the Judiciary on the Alleged Dye Monopoly*, 67th Congress, 1st session, 1922.

United States Congress, Senate, *Hearings Before the Subcommittee on Antitrust and Monopoly of the Committee of the Judiciary on Administered Prices*, 86th Congress, 2nd session, 1957.

PERIODICALS AND TECHNICAL JOURNALS

American Association of Pharmaceutical Chemists, Proceedings
American Journal of Pharmacy
American Journal of Syphilology and Chemotherapeutics
American Pharmaceutical Association, Proceedings
American Pharmaceutical Manufacturers' Association, Proceedings
Annales de l'Institut Pasteur
Annual Commercial Review of Philadelphia

Archives of Dermatology and Syphilology
Berlinische Klinische Wochenschrift
Boston Medical and Surgical Journal
Buffalo Medical and Surgical Journal
Chemist and Druggist
College and Clinical Record (Philadelphia)
College of Physicians of Philadelphia, Transactions
Deutsche Medicinische Wochenschrift
Dietetic and Hygiene Gazette
Drug and Cosmetic Review
Drug Industries Directories (Druggists Blue Book)
Drug Markets Catalogue and Directory
Drug Topics Red Book
Drug Trade Service
Druggists' Bulletin
Fortune
International Journal of Medicine and Surgery
Interstate Druggist
Journal of Bacteriology
Journal of Cutaneous Diseases
Journal of Industrial and Engineering Chemistry
Journal of Infectious Diseases
Journal of Pathology and Bacteriology
Journal of Pharmacology and Experimental Therapeutics
Journal of the American Medical Association
Journal of the American Pharmaceutical Association
Journal of the Medical Society of New Jersey
Keystone (Mulford Newsletter)
Klinische Jahrbuch (Jena)
Medical and Surgical Reporter (Philadelphia)
Medical Bulletin
Medical Life
Medical News (New York)
Medical News (Philadelphia)
Medical Record
Medical Register
Medical Times (Philadelphia)
Medical Times and Gazette (London)
Mittheilungen aus dem Kaiserlichen Gesundheitsamt
Monthly Cyclopedia and Medical Bulletin
Mulford Digest
New Remedies
New York City Board of Health, Annual Reports
New York City Board of Health, Monthly Bulletin
New York City Board of Health, Scientific Bulletin
New York Medical Journal
New York State Medical Association, Transactions
Northwestern Druggist
NSRD Journal

Parke Davis and Company, Annual Reports
Pennsylvania Pharmaceutical Association, Proceedings
Pennsylvania Medical Society, Transactions
Pennsylvania State Board of Health, Annual Reports
Pharmaceutical Era
Philadelphia Board of Health, Annual Reports
Philadelphia College of Pharmacy, Alumni Report
Philadelphia Medical Journal
Progress in Chemotherapy and the Treatment of Syphilis
Science
United States Marine Hospital and Public Health Service, Annual Reports
United States Marine Hospital and Public Health Service, Hygienic Laboratory
    Bulletins
United States Marine Hospital and Public Health Service, Public Health
    Reports
United States Patent Commission, Annual Reports
University (of Pennsylvania) *Medical Magazine*
Veterinary Bulletin (Mulford)
Veterinary Magazine of Philadelphia
Yearbook of Dermatology and Syphilology
Zeitschrift fuer Hygiene
Zeitschrift fuer Immunitaetsforschung und Experimentelle Therapie

OTHER PRIMARY SOURCES

Abbott, Alexander, *The Hygiene of Transmissible Diseases* (Philadelphia: Lea Brothers, 1909).

Andrews, F. W. *Diphtheria, Its Bacteriology, Pathology and Immunology* (London: HMSO, 1923).

Anon., *How to Succeed as a Physician, Heart to Heart Talks of a Successful Physician with his Brother Practitioners* (Meriden, Conn.: Church Publishing Co., 1902).

Ball, M. V., *Essentials of Bacteriology* (Philadelphia: Saunders, 1891).

Blodget, Lorin, *Census of Manufacturers of Philadelphia (1822)* (Philadelphia: Dickson and Gilling, 1883).

Bretonneau, P. F., *Des Inflammations Speciales du tissu Muqueux* (Paris: Crevot, 1826).

Committee on the Costs of Medical Care, *Medical Care for the American People* (Chicago: University of Chicago Press, 1932).

Crookshank, Edgar March, *An Introduction to Practical Bacteriology* (New York: Vail, 1886).

Dudgeon, Leonard Stanley, *Bacterial Vaccines and their Position in Therapeutics* (New York: Hoeber, 1927).

Ehrlich, Paul, *Collected Papers*, edited by F. Himmelweit, M. Marquardt and Sir H. Dale (London: Pergamon 1956–60).

Ehrlich, Paul, *Collected Studies on Immunity* (New York: Wiley, 1906).

Ehrlich, Paul, and Hata S., *Die Experimentelle Chemotherapie der Spirilossen* (Berlin: Springer, 1910).

Jordan, Edwin O., *A Text-Book of General Bacteriology* (Philadelphia: Saunders, 1908).

Flexner, Abraham, *Medical Education in the United States and Canada* (New York: Carnegie Foundation, 1910).

Kolle, W. (ed.) *Arbeiten aus den Staatsinstitut fuer Experimentelle Therapie und der Georg Speyer-Haus au Frankfurt a. M.* (Jena: Georg Speyer-Haus, 1927).

Lyons, Albert B., *Manual of Practical Pharmaceutical Assaying* (Detroit: Parke Davis, 1886).

The Merchant's Guide, *Philadelphia in 1800 and in 1907* (Philadelphia: Merchants and Travelers Association, 1907).

Philadelphia Board of Trade, *Manufacturers of Philadelphia, Census* (Philadelphia: Collins, 1861).

Pittinger, Paul S., *Biochemic Drug Assay Methods* (Philadelphia: Blakiston, 1914).

Rustby, Henry H., *Jungle Memories* (New York: Whittesey, 1933).

Seely, F. A., 'International Protection of Industrial Property', in *Proceedings and Addresses on the Patent System* (Washington, DC: Gedney and Roberts, 1892).

United States Bureau of the Census, *Census* (Washington, DC: USGPO, 1860–1920).

Waterbury, C. H., *How to Get It – Also Decisions Governing Distribution. A Manual for Manufacturers, Proprietors, Advertisers, Advertising Agencies and Buyers – Practical Answers to Practical Problems* (New York: National Wholesale Druggists' Association, 1923).

Wood, Horatio C., *A Treatise on Therapeutics* (Philadelphia: Lippincott, 1874).

Wood, Horatio C., Remington, J. R., and Sadler, S. P., *The Dispensatory of the United States of America* (Philadelphia: Lippincott, 1883).

SECONDARY SOURCES

Abbot, Alexander C., *The Development of Public Health Work in Philadelphia* (Philadelphia: 1909).

Abramovitz, Moses, 'Resources and Output Trends in the U.S. Since 1870', *American Economic Review*, 46 (1956) pp. 5–23.

Ackerknecht, Erwin H., *Therapeutics from the Primitives to the Twentieth Century* (New York: Hafner, 1973).

Adams, Walter (ed.) *The Structure of American Industry* (New York: Macmillan, 1977).

Aiken, Hugh, *Syntony and Spark. The Origins of Radio* (New York: Wiley, 1976).

American Foundation, *Medical Research: A Midcentury Survey* (Boston: Little, Brown, 1955).

American Pharmaceutical Association, *Brief History* (Washington, DC: American Pharmaceutical Association, 1949).

American Pharmaceutical Association, 'History and Summary of the Activities of the American Pharmaceutical Association', *Journal of the American Pharmaceutical Association*, Scientific edition 47, supplement 2–3 (1958).

Anderson, Oscar E., Jr, *The Health of a Nation. Harvery W. Wiley and the Fight for Pure Food* (Chicago: University of Chicago Press, 1950).

Apple, Rima B., '"To Be Used Only Under the Directions of a Physician": Commercial Infant Feeding and Medical Practice', *Bulletin of the History of Medicine*, 54 (1980) pp. 402–17.

Atwater, Edward C., 'The Medical Profession in a New Society', *Bulletin of the History of Medicine*, 51 (1977) pp. 93–106.

Bachmeyer, Arthur C., and Hartman, Gerrhard (eds) *The Hospital in Modern Society* (New York: Commonwealth Fund, 1943).

Bachmeyer, Arthur C., and Hartman, Gerrhard, *Hospital Trends and Developments 1940–1946* (New York: Commonwealth Fund, 1948).

Baltzell, E. Digby, *An American Business Aristocracy* (New York: Collier, 1962).

Baltzell, E. Digby, *Philadelphia Gentlemen. The Making of a National Upper Class* (Glencoe, Ill.: Free Press, 1958).

Baltzell, E. Digby, *Puritan Boston and Quaker Philadelphia* (New York: Basic Books, 1979).

Bealle, Morris A., *The Drug Story, a Factological History of America's $10,000,000,000 Drug Cartel. Its methods, operations, hidden ownership profits and . . . impact on the health of the American people* (Washington: Columbia Publications, 1950).

Bechet, Paul E., *A History of the American Dermatological Association in Commemoration of its Seventy-Fifth Anniversary, 1876–1951* (New York: Froben Press, 1952).

Beer, John J., 'Coal Tar Dye Manufacture and the Origins of the Modern Industrial Research Laboratory', *Isis*, 49 (1958) pp. 123–31.

Beer, John J., *The Origins of the German Chemical Industry*, (Urbana: University of Illinois Press, 1959).

Bender, George A., 'Henry Hurd Rusby', *Pharmacy in History*, 23 (1981) pp. 71–85.

Bentley, A. G., and Mumford, F. R., 'Developments in Pharmaceutical Apparatus', *Pharmaceutical Journal*, 146 (1941) pp. 148–51.

Bergey, David H., 'Early Instruction in Bacteriology in the United States', *American Medical History*, 1 (1917) pp. 426–7.

Berman, Alex, 'The Heroic Approach in 19th Century Therapeutics', *Bulletin of the American Society of Hospital Pharmacists* (1954) pp. 320–7.

Berman, Alex, *Pharmaceutical Historiography* (Madison, Wisconsin: American Institute for the History of Pharmacy, 1967).

Bernamann, W., 'Arzneimittelforschung and entwicklung in Deutschland in der zweiten halften des 19 jahrhunderte', *Pharmaceutische Industrie*, 29 (1967) pp. 448–9, 525–9, 669–73, 745–8, 834–6, 963–6, 1032–5.

Bett, W. R., 'From "dosimetric granules" to tridione, the briefly told story of Abbott Laboratories in Amercia', *Chemist and Druggist*, 168 (1957) p. 409.

Beyer, Karl H., *Discovery Development and Delivery of New Drugs* (New York: SP Medical and Scientific Books, 1978).

Birr, Kendall, *Pioneering Industrial Research* (Washington, DC: Public Affair Press, 1957).

Blake, John (ed.) *Safeguarding the Public* (Baltimore: Johns Hopkins University Press, 1974).

Blochman, Lawrence G., *Doctor Squibb, The Life and Times of a Rugged Individualist* (New York: Simon and Schuster, 1958).

Bonner, Thomas Neville, *American Doctors and German Universities. A Chapter in International Intellectual Relations, 1870–1914* (Nebraska: University of Nebraska Press, 1963).

Borell, Merriley, 'Setting the Standards for a New Science: Edward Schafner and Endocrinology', *Medical History*, 22 (1978) pp. 282–90.

Brieger, G., 'American Surgery and the Germ Theory of Disease', *Journal of History of Medicine*, 39 (1965) pp. 135–45.

Brieger, G., *Medical America in the Nineteenth Century* (Baltimore: Johns Hopkins University Press, 1972).

Brieger, G., 'Therapeutic Conflict and the American Medical Profession in the 1860s', *Bulletin of the History of Medicine*, 41 (1967) pp. 215–23.

Bulloch, William, *The History of Bacteriology* (New York: Dover, 1979).

Burlington, Robert, *The Odyssey of Modern Drug Research* (Kalamazoo, 1951).

Burrow, James G., *AMA: Voice of American Medicine* (Baltimore: Johns Hopkins University Press, 1963).

Bynum, William F., 'Chemical Structure and Pharmacological Action: A Chapter in the History of 19th Century Pharmacology', *Bulletin of the History of Medicine*, 44 (1970) pp. 518–38.

Carey, Eben James, *Medical Science Exhibits: A Century of Progress* (Chicago: Century of Progress Publishing, 1936).

Carter, K. Codell, 'The Germ Theory, Beriberi and the Deficiency Theory of Disease', *Medical History*, 21 (1977) pp. 119–36.

Chain, Ernest B., 'Academic and Industrial Contributions to Drug Research', *Nature*, 200 (1963) pp. 441–51.

Chandler, Alfred D., Jr, *The Visible Hand. The Managerial Revolution in American Business* (Cambridge, Mass.: Harvard University Press, 1977).

Chandler, Alfred D., Jr, and Daems, Herman, (eds) *Managerial Hierarchies: Comparative Perspectives on the Rise of the Modern Industrial Enterprise* (Cambridge, Mass.: Harvard University Press, 1980).

Chapman, Stanley, *Jesse Boot of Boots the Chemists: A Study in Business History* (London: Hodder and Stoughton, 1974).

CIBA Ltd, *The Story of Chemical Industry in Basle* (Lausanne: Graf, 1959).

Clark, Paul Franklin, *Pioneer Microbiologists of America* (Madison: University of Wisconsin Press, 1961).

Clark, Roscoe C., *Threescore Years and Ten. A History of Eli Lilly and Company* (Columbia: Lilly, 1964).

Clark, Victor S., *History of Manufacturers in the United States 1860–1914*, Vol. II (Washington, DC: Carnegie Institute of Washington, 1928).

Cochran, Thomas C., *Basic History of American Business* (Princeton: Van Nostrand, 1959).

Cochran, Thomas C., *American Business in the Twentieth Century* (Cambridge: Harvard University Press, 1972).

Cochran, Thomas C., *Business in American Life: A History* (New York: McGraw-Hill, 1972).

Cochran, Thomas C., and Miller, William, *The Age of Enterprise. A Social History of Industrial America* (New York: Macmillan, 1942).

Collins, H. M., 'The TEA Set: Tacit Knowledge and Scientific Networks', *Science Studies*, 4 (1874) pp. 164–86.

Comanor, William, 'The Drug Industry and Medical Research', *Journal of Business* (1966) pp. 12–18.

Compton, Walter Ames, *Serving Needs in Health and Nutrition* (New York: Newcomen Society in North America, 1973).

Cooper, Michael H., *Prices and Profits in the Pharmaceutical Industry* (Oxford: Pergamon Press, 1960).

Corner, George W., *A History of the Rockefeller Institute, 1901–1953 Origins and Growth* (New York: Rockefeller Institute Press, 1964).

Corner, George W., *Two Centuries of Medicine. A History of the School of Medicine, University of Pennsylvania* (Philadelphia: Lippincott, 1965).

Cowan, David L., 'The Role of the Pharmaceutical Industry', *Medical Sciences* (1970) pp. 72–82.

Coulter, Harris L., *Divided Legacy: A History of the Schism in Medical Thought* (Washington, DC: American Institute of Homeopathy, 1973).

Croskey, John W., *History of Blockley, A History of the Philadelphia General Hospital, 1731–1928* (Philadelphia: Davis, 1929).

Dean, R. L., 'How the Proposed Drug Regulation Reform Act Will Discourage the Search for New Drugs', *New England Journal of Medicine*, 299 (1978) pp. 413–15.

Dehaen P., 'Golden Years of Drug Introduction 1941–1970', *New York State Journal of Medicine*, 72 (1972) pp. 253–8.

Dixon, Bernard, *Beyond the Magic Bullet* (Boston: Allen and Unwin, 1978).

Dopson, Laurence, 'A Pioneer of Elegant Medicines. Dr Edmund Kirby and his Association with H. T. Kirby and Co. Ltd.', *Chemist and Druggist*, 168 (1957) pp. 538–9, 593–4.

Dowling, Harry F., *Fighting Infection: Conquests of the Twentieth Century* (Cambridge, Mass.: Harvard University Press, 1972).

Duckworth, Allen, 'Rise of the Pharmaceutical Industry', *Chemist and Druggist*, 100 (1959).

Duffy, John, *A History of Public Health in New York City 1866–1966* (New York: Russell Sage Foundation, 1974).

Dunlop, Sir Derrick, *Medicines in our Time* (London: Nuffield Provincial Hospitals Trust, 1973).

Dupree, A. Hunter, *Science in the Federal Government, A History of Policies and Achievements to 1940* (Cambridge, Mass.: Harvard University Press, 1957).

Eccles, J. C., and Gibson, William C., *Sherrington: His Life and Thought* (London: Springer International, 1979).

Edwards, Sir Ronald, 'The Multinational Pharmaceutical Industry: A Commentary', *Mercantile Credit Lecture* (London: Mercantile Credit, 1974).

Elder, Albert L., 'The History of Penicillin Production', *Chemical Engineering Progress Symposium Series*, 100, No. 66 (1975) pp. vi, 100.

Engel, Leonard, *Medicine Makers of Kalamazoo* (New York: McGraw-Hill, 1961).

England, Joseph W. (ed.) *The First Century of the Philadelphia College of*

Pharmacy, 1821–1921 (Philadelphia: Philadelphia College of Pharmacy, 1922).

Ernst and Ernst Company, *A History of the Firm* (Cleveland: Ernst and Ernst, 1960).

Evans Medical Supplies Ltd, *The Story of Evans Medical Supplies, 1809–1959* (Liverpool and London: Evans Medical Supplies, 1959).

Evans Medical Supplies Ltd, '150 Years of Progress – The Sesquicentenary of Evans Medical Ltd.', *Pharmaceutical Journal*, 183 pp. 61–2.

Fisher, Albert B., *Warehouse Operations of Service Wholesale Druggists* (Columbus: Ohio State University Press, 1918).

Fleming, Donald, *William H. Welch and the Rise of Modern Medicine* (Boston: Little, Brown, 1954).

Fleming, Grant, 'Canadian and British Experience in the Economics of Medical Practice', *College of Physicians of Philadelphia, Transactions*, 42 (1934) pp. 38–49.

Folk, G. F., *Patents and Industrial Progress* (New York: Harper, 1942).

Fox, Renee, 'Advanced Medical Technology, Social and Ethical Implications', *Annual Review of Sociology*, 2 (1976) pp. 231–68.

Friedman, Reuben (ed.) *A History of Dermatology in Philadelphia Including a Biography of Louis A. Duhring, M.D., Father of Dermatology in Philadelphia* (Fort Pierce Beach, Florida: Froben Press, 1955).

Frohlich, W., 'The Physician and the Pharmaceutical Industry in the United States', *Proceedings of the Royal Society of Medicine* (1955) pp. 579–86.

Galambos, Louis B., *The Public Image of Big Business in America 1880–1940. A Quantitative Study in Social Change* (Baltimore: Johns Hopkins University Press, 1975).

Gamble, F. H., and Evers, Norman, 'Advances in the Manufacture of Pharmaceutical Products', *Pharmaceutical Journal*, 134 (1935) pp. 541–3.

Garrison, Fielding H., *An Introduction to the History of Medicine*, 4th ed. (Philadelphia: Saunders, 1929).

Garrison, Fielding H., *John Shaw Billings, A Memoir* (New York: Putnam, 1915).

Geigy, 'Bicentenary of Geigy – The Group's History of Achievements', *Pharmaceutical Journal*, 180 (1958) p. 447.

General Advertising Company of London Ltd, *The History of Duncan Flockhart and Co. Commemorating the Centenaries of Ether and Chloroform* (Edinburgh: Duncan, Flockhart, 1947).

Gerhardt, O., 'The German Pharmaceutical Industry', *German Medical Monthly*, 6 (1961) pp. 94–6.

Grabowski, H. G., *Drug Regulation and Innovation* (Washington, DC: American Enterprise Institution, 1975).

Greenbaum, Sigmund S., and Wright, Carroll S., 'Memoir of J. Frank Schamberg', *Urologic and Cutaneous Review*, 51 (1947) pp. 251–3.

Greenberg, Danial S., 'Drug Regulation Reform', *New England Journal of Medicine*, 198 (1978) pp. 979–80.

Greenberg, Danial S., 'F.D.A.: A Miracle in Rockville', *New England Journal of Medicine*, 4, No. 298 (1978) pp. 227–8.

Greenwood, J. E., *A Cap for Boots: An Autobiography* (London: Hutchinson, 1977).

Griffenhagen, George B., and Romaine, Lawrence B., 'Early U.S. Pharmaceutical Catalogues', *American Journal of Pharmacy* (1959) pp. 14–33.

Groebli, Rene, 'A Name after the Chemical Industry Itself', *Ciba-Geigy Journal*, 1 (1971) pp. 26–33.

Haller, John S., Jr, 'Medical Theory of the Use and Abuse of Calomel in Nineteenth Century America', *Pharmacy in History*, 131 (1971) pp. 27–34, 67–76.

Haller, John S., Jr, 'The Use and Abuse of Tartar Emetic in the 19th Century Materia Medica', *Bulletin of the History of Medicine*, 49 (1975) pp. 235–57.

Hanbury, Sir John, 'A Reminiscence: Pharmacy in the First Half of the 20th Century', *Pharmaceutical History*, 8 (1978) p. 6.

Harris, Richard, *The Real Voice* (New York: Macmillan, 1964).

Harrod, Kathryn E., *Man of Courage. The Story of Dr. Edward L. Trudeau* (New York: J. Messner, 1959).

Harvey, A. McGehee, 'John Billings: Forgotten Hero of American Medicine', *Perspectives on Biology and Medicine*, 21 (1978) pp. 353–7.

Hastings, E. G., and Morrey, C. B., 'Early Instructions in Bacteriology in the United States', *Journal of Bacteriology*, 3 (1978) pp. 307–8.

Haynes, Williams, *The American Chemical Industry: A History*, 6 vols (New York: Van Nostrand, 1945–52).

Hektoen, Ludvig, 'Notes on the History of Bacteriology in Chicago', *Bulletin of the Society for Medical History, Chicago*, 5 (1937) pp. 3–21.

Helfand, W. H., Woodruff, H. B., Coleman, K. M. H., and Cowen, D. L., 'Wartime Industrial Development of Penicillin in the United States', in John Parascandola (ed.) *The History of Antibiotics, a Symposium* (Madison: American Institute of the History of Pharmacy, 1980).

Hickel, E., *Arzneimittel-Standardisierung in 19. Jahrhundert in den Pharmakopoen Deutschlands, Frankreichs, Grossbritanniens und der Vereinigten Staaten von Amerika.* (Stuttgart: Wisenschafftlische Verlassgesellschafft, 1973).

Hill, Charles Alexander, 'The Changing Foundations of Pharmaceutical Manufacture', *Pharmaceutical Journal*, 134 (1935) pp. 533–5.

Horns, Seymour E., *Economics of American Medicine* (New York: Macmillan, 1964).

Hudson, Robert P., 'Abraham Flexner in Perspective: American Medical Education 1865–1904', *Bulletin of the History of Medicine*, 46 (1972) pp. 545–61.

Huisking, Charles L., *Herbs to Hormones. The Evolution of Drugs and Chemicals that Revolutionized Medicine* (Connecticut: Pequot Press, 1968).

Inglis, Brian, *Drugs, Doctors and Disease* (London: Andre Deutsch, 1965).

International Record of Medical and General Practice, 'Ten Years' Experience With Diphtheria Antitoxin', *New York Medical Journal*, 82 (1905).

Jackson, Charles O., *Food and Drug Legislation in the New Deal* (Princeton: Princeton University Press, 1970).

Jackson, Charles O., 'Muckraking and Consumer Protection. The Case of the 1938 Food, Drug and Cosmetic Act', *Pharmacy in History*, 13 (1971) pp. 103–10.

Jenkins, Reese V., *Images and Enterprise: Technology and the American Photographic Industry 1839–1935* (Baltimore: Johns Hopkins University

Press, 1975).

Kahn, E. J., *All in a Century . . . the First 100 years of Eli Lilly and Co.* (Indianapolis: Eli Lilly, 1976).

Keele, C. A. 'Empiricism and Logic in the Discovery of New Drugs', *Nature*, 195 (1962) p. 642.

Kendall, Henry P., *The Kendall Company, Fifty Years of Yankee Enterprise* (New York: The Newcomen Society in North America, 1953).

Kennedy, Donald, 'Creative Tension: FDA and Medicine', *New England Journal of Medicine*, 298 (1978) pp. 846–50.

Kett, Joseph F., *The Formation of the American Medical Profession. The Role of Institutions, 1780–1860* (New Haven: Yale University Press).

Kolmer, J. A., 'The History of Laboratory Research in the Past Fifty Years', *Medical Life*, 34 (1927) pp. 3–14.

Kogan, Herman, *The Long White Line. The Story of Abbott Laboratories* (New York: Random House, 1963).

Kramer, H. D., 'The Germ Theory and the Early Public Health Program in the United States', *Bulletin of the History of Medicine*, 22 (1948) p. 241.

Kremers, Edward and Urdang, George, *History of Pharmacy*, 4th ed. (Philadelphia: Lippincott, 1976).

Lardon, R. L. (ed.) *Regulating New Drugs* (Chicago: University of Chicago Press, 1973).

Lasagna, Louis, 'The Development and Regulation of New Medications', *Science*, 200 (1978) pp. 871–3.

Lasagna, Louis, 'Research, Regulation and Development of New Pharmaceuticals: Past, Present, and Future – Part II', *American Journal of Medical Science*, 263 (1970) p. 70.

Lazell, Henry George, *From Pills to Penicillin: The Beecham Story: A Personal Account* (London: Heinemann, 1975).

Lee, Charles O., 'The Shakers as Pioneers in the American Herbal and Drug Industry', *American Journal of Pharmacy* 132 (1960) pp. 178–93.

Lewis, Sinclair, *Martin Arrowsmith* (London: Jonathan Cape, 1925).

Litchtin, A., and Schamberg, Ira Leo, 'Jay Frank Schamberg. A Pioneer in Dermatologic Research and Chemotherapy', *AMA Archives of Dermatology*, 73 (1956) p. 493.

Loyd, Harry J., *Parke-Davis, the Never-Ending Search for Better Medicines* (New York: Newcomen Society in North America, 1957).

McClung, L. S., 'The American Society for Microbiology/Society of American Bacteriologists: A Brief History', *American Society of Microbiology News*, 44 (1978) pp. 446–51.

McFarland, Joseph, 'The Beginning of Bacteriology in Philadelphia', *Bulletin of the History of Medicine*, 5 (1935) pp. 148–72.

Macfarlane, John James, *Manufacturing in Philadelphia 1683–1912* (Philadelphia: Community Museum, 1912).

Mahoney, John Thomas, *The Merchants of Life. An Account of the American Pharmaceutical Industry* (New York: Harper, 1959).

Maltbie, Birdsey Lucius, *A Quarter Century of Progress in Manufacturing Pharmacy* (New York: American Pharmaceutical Manufacturing Association, 1937).

Marion, John F., *The Fine Old House, The History of SmithKline Corp.*

(Philadelphia: SmithKline, 1980).

Marquardt, Maria, *Paul Ehrlich* (London: Permagon, 1949).

Mazumdar, P., 'The Antigen–Antibody Reaction and the Physics and Chemistry of Life', *Bulletin of the History of Medicine*, 48 (1974) pp. 1–21.

Measday, Walter, 'Pharmaceutical Industry', in Adams, Walter (ed.) *The Structure of American Industry* (New York: Macmillan, 1977).

Merck, Sharp and Dohme, *By Their Fruits: Some Historical Contributions to the Chemistry of Life* (Rahway, NJ: Merck, 1962).

Merck, A. G., *From Merck's Angel Pharmacy to the World Wide Merck Group 1668–1968* (Darmstadt: E. Merck, 1968).

Merrill, Lynch, Pierce, Fenner & Smith. *Chemical Industry Survey* (New York: Merrill Lynch, 1943).

Merwin, Samuel, *Rise and Fight Again: The Story of a Life Long Friend* (New York: Allen & Charlesborn, 1953).

Miles, Samuel, *Pfizer, An Informal History* (New York: Pfizer, 1978).

Mintz, Morton *The Therapeutic Nightmare* (Boston: Houghton Miffin, 1965).

Modell, W., 'Clinical Pharmacology: Reflections in my Rear-View Mirror', *Clinical Pharmacy and Therapeutics*, 23 (1978) pp. 497–504.

Moellers, Bernhard, *Robert Koch, Personenlichkeit, und Lebenswerk, 1843–1910* (Hannover: Schnell, 1950).

Morrison, Elting, *From Nowhere to Know How* (Cambridge, Mass.: MIT Press, 1976).

Muir, Ross L., *Over the Long Term: The Story of J. W. Seligman and Co. 1864–1964* (New York: J. W. Seligman and Co., 1964).

Munch, James C., and J. C., Jr, 'Notices of Judgement. The First Thousand', *Food Drug Cosmetic Law Journal*, 10 (1955) pp. 219–42.

National Wholesale Druggists Association, *A History of the National Wholesale Druggists' Association From its Organization to 1924. Half a Century of Constructive Service* (National Wholesale Druggists Association, 1924).

Navin, Thomas R., and Sears, Marian V., 'The Rise of a Market for Industrial Securities, 1887–1902', *Business History Review*, 23 (1955) pp. 105–38.

Neisser, A., 'On Modern Syphiliotherapy, with Particular Reference to Salvarsan', *Bulletin of the History of Medicine*, 16 (1944) pp. 469–510.

Noble, David F., *America By Design: Science, Technology and the Rise of Corporate Capitalism* (New York: Knopf, 1977).

Noyes Data Corporation, *Pharmaceutical and Cosmetic Firms, U.S.A., 1970* (Park Ridge, NJ: Noyes Data Corp., 1970).

Numbers, Ronald (ed.) *The Education of American Physicians* (Berkeley: University of California Press 1980).

Oliver, Wayde W., *The Man Who Lived for Tomorrow. William Hallock Park* (New York: Dutton, 1941).

Olsen, P. C., *The Merchandising of Drug Products* (New York: Appleton, 1931).

Parish, Henry James, *Victory with Vaccines: The Story of Immunization* (Edinburgh: Livingstone, 1968).

Parke Davis, *Parke-Davis at 100. Progress in the Past . . . Promise For the Future. 1866–1966 100th Anniversary* (Detroit: Parke Davis, 1966).

Parke Davis, *Scientific Contributions from the Laboratories 1866–1966* (Detroit: Parke Davis, 1966).

Pelmer, Louis, 'Jay Frank Schomberg, M.D., (1870–1934). Medical Scholar and Founder of the Independent American Pharmaceutical Industry', *Medical Times*, 97 (1968) pp. 95–100.

Pennsylvania Pharmaceutical Association, *A History of the Activities of the Pennsylvania Pharmaceutical Association, 1878–1978* (Pittsburgh: Pennsylvania Pharmaceutical Association, 1978).

Pfizer (Charles) and Company, *Then – 1849, and Now – 1959: A Century and a Decade of Progress* (New York: Charles Pfizer and Co., 1960).

Porter, Glenn, *The Rise of Big Business 1860–1910* (New York: Collins, 1976).

Porter, Glenn, and Livesay, Harold C., *Merchants and Manufacturers: Studies in the Changing Structure of Nineteenth Century Marketing* (Baltimore: Johns Hopkins University Press, 1974).

Reiser, Stanley Joel, *Medicine and the Reign of Technology* (Cambridge: Cambridge University Press, 1978).

B. C. Remedy Company, *B. C. 50th Anniversary* (Durham: B. C. Remedy Co., n.d.).

Reverby, Susan, and Rosner, David (eds) *Health Care in America, Essays in Social History* (Philadelphia: Temple University Press, 1979).

Rexell Drug Company, *The Story of Rexell Drug Co.* (Los Angeles: Rexell Drug Co.).

Richmond, P. Allen, 'Some Variant Theories in Opposition to the Germ Theory of Disease', *Journal of the History of Medicine and Allied Sciences*, 4 (1954) pp. 290–303.

Richmond, P. Allen, 'American Attitudes toward the Germ Theory of Disease (1860–1880)', *Journal of the History of Medicine and Allied Sciences*, 9 (1959) pp. 428–54.

Risse, Guenter B., 'The Renaissance of Bloodletting: A Chapter in Modern Therapeutics', *Journal of the History of Medicine and Allied Sciences*, 34 (1979) pp. 3–22.

Risse, Guenter B., 'The Brownian System of Medicine: Its Theoretical and Practical Implications', *Clio Medica*, 5 (1970) pp. 45–51.

Risse, Guenter B., Numbers, R. L. and Leavitt, J. W. (eds) *Medicine Without Doctors, Home Health Care in American History* (New York: Science History Publishers, 1977).

Rorem, C. R., and Fischelis, R. P., *The Costs of Medicine* (Chicago: Committee on the Costs of Medical Care, 1932).

Rosen G., 'Patterns of Health Research in the United States 1900–1960', *Bulletin of the History of Medicine*, 39 (1965) pp. 201–21.

Rosen G., *Fees and Fee Bills* (Baltimore: Johns Hopkins University Press, 1946).

Rosen G., *From Medical Police to Social Medicine: Essays on the History of Health Care* (New York: Science History Publishers, 1974).

Rosen G., *Preventive Medicine in the United States 1900–1975* (New York: Science History Publishers, 1975).

Rosen, G., *History of Public Health* (New York: M.D. Publications, 1958).

Rosenberg, Charles, E., *No Other Gods. On Science and American Social Thought* (Baltimore, Johns Hopkins University Press, 1978).

Rosengren, William R., and Lefton, Mark, *Hospitals and Patients* (New York:

Atherton, 1969).

Rosenkrantz, Barbara G., *Public Health and the State. Changing Views in Massachusetts 1842–1936* (Cambridge, Mass.: Harvard University Press, 1972).

Roth, Julius A., *Health Purifiers and Their Enemies* (New York: Neil Watson, 1977).

Rothstein, William, *American Physicians in the Nineteenth Century, from Sects to Science* (Baltimore: Johns Hopkins University Press, 1972).

Rubenstein, William D., *Men of Property* (London: Croom Helm, 1981).

Ryan, K. J., 'The FDA and the Practice of Medicine', *New England Journal of Medicine*, 297 (1975) pp. 1287–8.

Scharf, John T., and Westcott, Thompson, *History of Philadelphia 1609–1804* (Philadelphia: Little Evans, 1884).

Schiefflin and Company, *One Hundred Years of Business Life, 1794–1894* (New York: Schiefflin, 1894).

Schieffelin & Company, *150 Years of Service to American Health* (New York: Schiefflin, 1944).

Schmeckebier, Lawrence F., *The Public Health Service. Its History, Activities and Organization* (Baltimore: Johns Hopkins University Press, 1923).

Schneider, Wolfgang, *Geschichte der Deutschen Pharmazeutischen Gesellschaft 1890–1965* (Munchen: Verlag Chemie, 1965).

Schwartzman, E., *Innovation in the Pharmaceutical Industry* (Baltimore: Johns Hopkins University Press, 1976).

Shaw, Robert B., *History of the Comstock Patent Medicine Business and Dr. Morse's Indian Root Pills* (Washington, DC: Smithsonian Institution Press, 1972).

Sherrington, Charles, 'Sir Charles Sherrington's First Use of Diphtheria Antitoxin Made in England', *Notes and Records of the Royal Society of London*, 4 (1946) pp. 156–9.

Shryock, Richard M., *American Medical Research Past and Present* (New York: Commonwealth Fund, 1957).

Shryock, Richard M., *The Development of Modern Medicine: An Interpretation of the Social and the Scientific Factors Involved* (New York: Hafner Publisher, 1969).

Sinclair, Upton, *The Jungle*, New York: Signet, 1960.

Silverman, Milton, and Lee, Philip R., *Pills, Profits and Politics* (Berkeley: University of California Press, 1974).

Smith, George Winston, *Medicines for the Union Army* (Madison: American Institute for the History of Pharmacy, 1962).

Smith, George Winston, 'The Squibb Laboratory in 1863', *Journal of the History of Medicine and Allied Sciences*, 13 (1958) pp. 382–94.

Spink, Wesley W., *Infectious Diseases. Prevention and Treatment in the Nineteenth and Twentieth Centuries* (Folkestone, Kent: Dawson, 1978).

Sonnedecker, Glenn, 'The Rise of Drug Manufacture in America', *Emory University Quarterly*, 21 (1965) pp. 73–87.

Sonnedecker, Glenn, 'The Pharmacopeia and America – 150 Years of Service', *Pharmacy in History*, 12 (1970) pp. 156–69.

Squibb, E. R. and Sons, 'The House that Squibb built is This Year Celebrating the 100th Anniversary of Its Founding', *American Pharmaceutical Associa-*

198   *Bibliography*

tion, 16 (1958) pp. 616–7.

Stechl, Peter, 'The Biological Standardization of Drugs: The Origin of Probit Analysis', *Pharmacy in History*, 12 (1970) p. 145.

Steele, Henry, 'Monopoly and Competition in the Ethical Drug Market', *The Journal of Law and Economics* (1962) pp. 131–62.

Sterling, Drug Incorporated, *The Sterling Story* (New York: Sterling Drug Inc., n.d.).

Stevens, Rosemary, *American Medicine and the Public Interest* (New Haven: Yale University Press, 1971).

Strickland, Stephen P., *Politics, Science and Dread Disease. A Short History of United States Medical Research Policy* (Cambridge, Mass.: Harvard University Press, 1972).

Tainter, M. L., and Marcelli, G.M.A., 'The Rise of Synthetic Drugs in the American Pharmaceutical Industry', *Bulletin of the New York Academy of Medicine*, 35 (1959) pp. 387–405.

Taylor, F. O., 'Parke-Davis & Co.', *Industrial and Engineering Chemistry*, 19 (1927) pp. 1209.

Taylor, F. O., 'They Made Drug Therapy Reliable', *Therapeutic Notes* (1941) pp. 184–7.

Taylor, F. O., 'Forty-Five Years of Manufacturing Pharmacy', *Journal of the American Pharmaceutical Association*, 4 (1915) p. 471.

Taylor, Lloyd C., *The Medical Profession and Social Reform, 1885–1945* (New York: St Martin's, 1974).

Temin, Peter, *Taking Your Medicine. Drug Regulation in the United States* (Cambridge, Mass.: Harvard University Press, 1980).

Temkin, Oswei, 'Historical Aspects of Drug Therapy', in Paul Talalay (ed.) *Drugs in Our Society* (Baltimore: Johns Hopkins University Press, 1964) pp. 3–16.

Tishler, M., 'Role of the Drug House in Biological and Medical Research', *Bulletin of the New York Academy of Medicine*, 35 (1959) pp. 590–600.

United States Patent Office, *Development and Use of Patent Classification Systems* (Washington, DC: USGPO, 1966).

United States Patent Office, *Manual and Classification of Subjects of Invention of the U.S. Patent Office* (Washington, DC: USGPO, 1912).

Vallery-Radot, Rene, *The Life of Pasteur* (New York: Sun Dial Press, 1937).

Vogt, D. D., and Billups, N.F., 'The Merger Movement in the American Pharmaceutical Complex', *Journal of the American Pharmaceutical Association*, 11 (1971) pp. 588–91.

Vick Chemical Company, *Vick Builds for the Future: The Story of the Growth of a Diversified Drug Business* (New York: Vick Chemical Co., n.d.).

Waksman, Selman A., *My Life with the Mocribes* (London: Scientific Book Club, 1958).

Walker, Nona, *Medicine Makers* (New York: Hastings House, 1966).

Warner, John Harley, '"The Nature-Trusting Heresy": American Physicians and the Concept of the Healing Power of Nature in the 1850s and 1860s', *Perspectives in American History*, 11 (1977–1978) pp. 298–324.

Warner, John Harley, 'Physiological Theory and Therapeutic Explanation in the 1860s: The British Debate on the Medical Use of Alcohol', *Bulletin of the History of Medicine*, 54 (1980) pp. 235–57.

Warner, John Harley, 'Therapeutic Explanation and the Edinburgh Blood-letting Controversy: Two Perspectives on the Medical Meaning of Science in the Mid-Nineteenth Century', *Medical History*, 14 (1980) pp. 241–58.

Waserman, Manfred, 'The Quest for a National Health Department in the Progressive Era', *Bulletin of the History of Medicine*, 49 (1975) pp. 353–80.

Waterbury, C. H., *How to Get It* (New York: National Wholesale Druggists' Association, 1923).

Welch, William, 'The Evolution of Modern Scientific Laboratories', *Bulletin of Johns Hopkins Hospital*, 7 (1896) pp. 19–24.

Wiebe, Robert, *The Search for Order, 1877–1920* (New York: Hill and Wang, 1967).

Wiebe, Robert, *Businessmen and Reform: A Study of the Progressive Movement* (Cambridge, Mass.: Harvard University Press, 1962).

Wilbert, M. I., *Changes in the Pharmacopoeia and the National Formulary* (Washington, DC: USGPO, 1917).

Wilkinson, Herbert S., 'History and Evolution of Pharmaceutical Industry', *Journal of the American Pharmaceutical Industry*, 20 (1959) p. 592.

Williams, Ralph Chester, *The United States Public Health Service, 1798–1950* (Washington DC: Commissioned Officers' Association of the US Public Health Service, 1951).

Winslow, C. E. A., *The Life of Herman M. Biggs. Physician and Statesman of Public Health* (Philadelphia: Lea and Febiger, 1929).

Winslow, C. E. A., *The Conquest of Epidemic Disease.* (Princeton: Princeton University Press, 1943).

Wolfe, Margaret Ripley, *Lucius Polk Brown and Progressive Food and Drug Control: Tennessee and New York City, 1908–1920* (Lawrence: Regents Press of Kansas, 1978).

Woolf, Patricia, 'The Second Messinger: Informal Communication in Cyclic AMP Research', *Minerva*, 14 (1976) pp. 349–73.

Young, James Harvey, *The Toadstool Millionaires: A Social History of Patent Medicines in America Before Federal Regulation* (Princeton: Princeton University Press, 1961).

Young, James Harvey, *Medical Messiahs: A Social History of Health Quackery in Twentieth-Century America* (Princeton: Princeton University Press, 1967).

Young, James Harvey, *American Self-Dosage Medicines. An Historical Perspective* (Lawrence: Coronado, 1974).

Zeiss, H., and Bieling, B., *Behring, Gestalt und Werk* (Berlin: Schultz, 1941).

General Index

Index of Names

Index of Companies